Case No. _____

Veterinary Patient Organizer / SOAP Notebook /
History & Physical Exam Templates

By. Lance Wheeler

Case No. _____

By. Lance Wheeler

Property of: _____

Phone No.: _____

Date: _____

Table of Contents

Patient	Age	Sex	Breed	Weight
	DOB:	Mn / Mi Fs / Fi	Color:	kg

Owner	Primary Veterinarian	Admit Date/ Time
Name: Phone:	Name: Phone:	Date: Time: AM / PM

• **Presenting Complaint**:_____
_____
_____

• **Medical Hx**:_____
_____
_____

• **When/ where obtained**:   Date:_____;   ☐Breeder, ☐Shelter, Other:_____

Drug/ Suppl.	Amount	Dose (mg/kg)	Route	Frequency	Date Started

• **Vaccine status – Dog**: ☐Rab ☐Parv ☐Dist ☐Aden; ☐Para ☐Lep ☐Bord ☐Influ ☐Lyme
• **Vaccine status – Cat**: ☐Rab ☐Herp ☐Cali ☐Pan ☐FeLV[kittens]; ☐FIV ☐Chlam ☐Bord
• **Heartworm / Flea & Tick / Intestinal Parasites**:
   ◦ *Last Heartworm Test*: Date:_____, ☐IDK; Test Results: ☐Pos, ☐Neg, ☐IDK
   ◦ *Monthly heartworm preventative*:   ☐no ☐yes, Product:_____
   ◦ *Monthly flea & tick preventative*:   ☐no ☐yes, Product:_____
   ◦ *Monthly dewormer*:   ☐no ☐yes, Product:_____
• **Surgical Hx**: ☐Spay/Neuter; Date:_____; Other:_____
• **Environment**: ☐Indoor, ☐Outdoor, Time spent outdoors/ Other:_____
• **Housemates**: Dogs:_____ Cats:_____ Other:_____
• **Diet**: ☐Wet, ☐Dry; Brand/ Amt.:_____

Appetite	☐Normal, ☐↑, ☐↓
Weight	☐Normal, ☐↑, ☐↓; Past Wt.:_____ kg; Date:_____; Δ:_____
Thirst	☐Normal, ☐↑, ☐↓
Urination	☐Normal, ☐↑, ☐↓, ☐Blood, ☐Strain
Defecation	☐Normal, ☐↑, ☐↓, ☐Blood, ☐Strain, ☐Diarrhea, ☐Mucus
Discharge	☐No, ☐Yes; Onset/ Describe:
Cough/ Sneeze	☐No, ☐Yes; Onset/ Describe:
Vomit	☐No, ☐Yes; Onset/ Describe:
Respiration	☐Normal, ☐↑ Rate, ☐↑ Effort
Energy level	☐Normal, ☐Lethargic, ☐Exercise intolerance

• **Travel Hx**: ☐None, Other:_____
• **Exposure to**: ☐Standing water, ☐Wildlife, ☐Board/daycare, ☐Dog park, ☐Groomer
• **Adverse reactions to food/ meds**: ☐None, Other:_____
• **Can give oral meds**: ☐no ☐yes; Helpful Tricks:_____

Physical Exam – General:

- **Body Weight**:_____kg   **Body Condition Score**:_____/9

- **Temperature**:_____°F [*Dog-RI*: 100.9–102.4; *Cat-RI*: 98.1–102.1]

- **Heart**:
  - *Rate*:_____beats/min [Dog-RI: 60–180; Cat-RI: 140–240 (in hospital)]
  - *Rhythm*: ☐Regular, ☐Irregular
  - *Sounds*: ☐None, ☐Split sound, ☐Gallop, ☐Murmur, ☐Muffled
    - *Grade*: ☐1–2[soft, only at PMI], ☐3–4[moderate, mild radiate], ☐5–6[strong radiate, thrill]
    - *Timing*: ☐Systolic, ☐Diastolic, ☐Continuous
    - *PMI*:

	PMI	Over	Anatomic Boundaries
☐	Lt. apex	Mitral valve	5th to 6th ICS at level of CCJ
☐	Lt. base	Ao + Pul outflow	2nd to 4th ICS above the CCJ
☐	Rt. midheart	Tricuspid valve	3rd to 5th ICS near the CCJ
☐	Rt. sternal border	Right ventricle	5th to 7th ICS immediately dorsal to the sternum
☐	Sternal (cat)	Sternum	In cats, PMI offers very little clinical significance.

-     •   *Vertebral Heart Size*: Dog = 8.7–10.5; Cat = 6.9–8.1 (from cranial edge of T4)
-     •   *Innocent Murmur*: Grade 1-2, systolic, left base location, disappear by ~4 months of age, absent clinical signs

- **Pulses**:
  - *Pulse rate*:_____pulses/min
  - *Character*: ☐Sync, ☐Async; ☐Normokinetic, ☐Hyper-, ☐Hypo-, ☐Variable

- **Lungs**:
  - *Respiratory rate*:_____breaths/min [*RI*: 16–30]
  - *Depth/Effort*: ☐Norm, ☐Pant, ☐Deep, ☐Shallow, ☐↑ Insp effort, ☐↑ Exp effort
  - *Sounds/Localization*:
    - ☐Norm BV, ☐Quiet BV, ☐Loud BV, ☐Crack, ☐Wheez, ☐Frict, ☐Muffled
    - ☐All fields, ☐Rt cran, ☐Rt mid, ☐Rt caud, ☐Lt cran, ☐Lt mid, ☐Lt caud
  - *Tracheal Auscultation/ Palpation*: ☐Normal, Other:_____

- **Pain Score**:_____ / 5   Localization:_____

- **Mentation**: ☐BAR   ☐Confused/   ☐Drowsy/   ☐Stuporous   ☐Coma
                    ☐QAR   Disoriented   Obtunded   (unresponsive
                    ☐Dull   unless aroused by
                                                                 noxious stimuli)

- **Skin Elasticity**: ☐Normal skin turgor, ☐↓ Skin turgor, ☐Skin tent, ☐Gelatinous

- **Mucus Membranes**:
  - *CRT*:_____ [*RI*: 1–2; <1 = compensated shock, sepsis, heat stroke; <2 = acute decompensated shock; >2 = late decompensated shock, decreased cardiac output, hypothermia]
  - *Color*:_____ [*RI*: pink; red = compensated shock, sepsis, heat stroke; pale/white = anemia, shock; blue = cyanosis; yellow = hepatic disease, extravascular hemolysis; brown = met-Hb]
  - *Texture*:_____ [*RI*: moist = hydrated; tacky-to-dry = 5–12% dehydrated]

Physical Exam – Systems Checklist:

- Head:_____ ☐NAF
  - Ears: ☐Debris (mild / mod / sev) (AS / AD / AU),_____ ☐NAF
  - Eyes:_____ ☐NAF
    - Retinal:_____ ☐NAF

	→ ⓛ		ⓡ		ⓛ		ⓡ ←
☐	Normal Direct	☐	Normal Indirect	☐	Normal Indirect	☐	Normal Direct
☐	Abnormal Direct	☐	Abnormal Indirect	☐	Abnormal Indirect	☐	Abnormal Direct

  - Nose:_____ ☐NAF
  - Oral cavity: ☐Tarter/Gingivitis (mild / mod / sev),_____ ☐NAF
  - Mandibular lnn.: ☐Enlarged Lt., ☐Enlarged Rt.,_____ ☐NAF

- Neck:_____ ☐NAF
  - Superficial cervical lnn.: ☐Enlarged Lt., ☐Enlarged Rt.,___ ☐NAF
  - Thyroid:_____ ☐NAF

- Thoracic limb:_____ ☐NAF
  - Foot pads:_____ ☐NAF
  - Knuckling:_____ ☐NAF
  - Axillary lnn. [normally absent]:_____ ☐NAF

- Thorax:_____ ☐NAF

- Abdomen:_____ ☐NAF
  - Mammary chain:_____ ☐NAF
  - Penis/ Testicles/ Vulva:_____ ☐NAF
  - Superficial inguinal lnn. [normally absent]:_____ ☐NAF

- Pelvic limb:_____ ☐NAF
  - Foot pads:_____ ☐NAF
  - Knuckling:_____ ☐NAF
  - Popliteal lnn.: ☐Enlarged Lt., ☐Enlarged Rt.,_____ ☐NAF

- Skin:_____ ☐NAF
- Tail:_____ ☐NAF
- Rectal☞☉:_____ ☐NAF

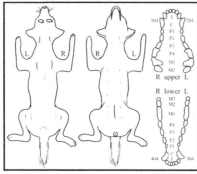

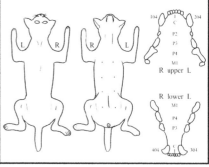

Problems List:

• **Problem #1**:

• **Problem #2**:

• **Problem #3**:

• **Problem #4**:

• **Problem #5**:

Diagnostic Plan	Treatment Plan

Patient	Age	Sex	Breed	Weight
	DOB:	Mn / Mi Fs / Fi	Color:	kg

Owner	Primary Veterinarian	Admit Date/ Time
Name: Phone:	Name: Phone:	Date: Time: AM / PM

• **Presenting Complaint**:_____
_____
_____

• **Medical Hx**:_____
_____
_____

• **When/ where obtained**:   Date:_____ ; □Breeder, □Shelter, Other:_____

Drug/ Suppl.	Amount	Dose (mg/kg)	Route	Frequency	Date Started

• **Vaccine status – Dog**: □Rab □Parv □Dist □Aden; □Para □Lep □Bord □Influ □Lyme
• **Vaccine status – Cat**: □Rab □Herp □Cali □Pan □FeLV[kittens]; □FIV □Chlam □Bord
• **Heartworm / Flea & Tick / Intestinal Parasites**:
  ◦ *Last Heartworm Test*: Date:_____, □IDK; Test Results: □Pos, □Neg, □IDK
  ◦ *Monthly heartworm preventative*: □no □yes, Product:_____
  ◦ *Monthly flea & tick preventative*: □no □yes, Product:_____
  ◦ *Monthly dewormer*:   □no □yes, Product:_____
• **Surgical Hx**:   □Spay/Neuter; Date:_____; Other:_____
• **Environment**: □Indoor, □Outdoor, Time spent outdoors/ Other:_____
• **Housemates**: Dogs:_____ Cats:_____ Other:_____
• **Diet**: □Wet, □Dry; Brand/ Amt.:_____

Appetite	□Normal, □↑, □↓
Weight	□Normal, □↑, □↓; Past Wt.:_____ kg; Date:_____; Δ:_____
Thirst	□Normal, □↑, □↓
Urination	□Normal, □↑, □↓, □Blood, □Strain
Defecation	□Normal, □↑, □↓, □Blood, □Strain, □Diarrhea, □Mucus
Discharge	□No, □Yes; Onset/ Describe:
Cough/ Sneeze	□No, □Yes; Onset/ Describe:
Vomit	□No, □Yes; Onset/ Describe:
Respiration	□Normal, □↑ Rate, □↑ Effort
Energy level	□Normal, □Lethargic, □Exercise intolerance

• **Travel Hx**: □None, Other:_____
• **Exposure to**: □Standing water, □Wildlife, □Board/daycare, □Dog park, □Groomer
• **Adverse reactions to food/ meds**: □None, Other:_____
• **Can give oral meds**: □no □yes; Helpful Tricks:_____

Physical Exam – General:

• **Body Weight**:_____kg   **Body Condition Score**:_____/9

• **Temperature**:_____°F [*Dog-RI*: 100.9–102.4; *Cat-RI*: 98.1–102.1]

• **Heart**:
  - *Rate*:_____beats/min [Dog-RI: 60–180; Cat-RI: 140–240 (in hospital)]
  - *Rhythm*: □Regular, □Irregular
  - *Sounds*: □None, □Split sound, □Gallop, □Murmur, □Muffled
    - *Grade*: □1–2[soft, only at PMI], □3–4[moderate, mild radiate], □5–6[strong radiate, thrill]
    - *Timing*: □Systolic, □Diastolic, □Continuous
    - *PMI*:

	PMI	Over	Anatomic Boundaries
□	Lt. apex	Mitral valve	5th to 6th ICS at level of CCJ
□	Lt. base	Ao + Pul outflow	2nd to 4th ICS above the CCJ
□	Rt. midheart	Tricuspid valve	3rd to 5th ICS near the CCJ
□	Rt. sternal border	Right ventricle	5th to 7th ICS immediately dorsal to the sternum
□	Sternal (cat)	Sternum	In cats, PMI offers very little clinical significance.

  - *Vertebral Heart Size*: Dog = 8.7–10.5; Cat = 6.9–8.1 (from cranial edge of T4)
  - *Innocent Murmur*: Grade 1-2, systolic, left base location, disappear by ~4 months of age, absent clinical signs

• **Pulses**:
  - *Pulse rate*:_____pulses/min
  - *Character*: □Sync, □Async; □Normokinetic, □Hyper-, □Hypo-, □Variable

• **Lungs**:
  - *Respiratory rate*:_____breaths/min [*RI*: 16–30]
  - *Depth/Effort*: □Norm, □Pant, □Deep, □Shallow, □↑ Insp effort, □↑ Exp effort
  - *Sounds/Localization*:
    - □Norm BV, □Quiet BV, □Loud BV, □Crack, □Wheez, □Frict, □Muffled
    - □All fields, □Rt cran, □Rt mid, □Rt caud, □Lt cran, □Lt mid, □Lt caud
  - *Tracheal Auscultation/ Palpation*: □Normal, Other:_____

• **Pain Score**:_____ / 5   Localization:_____

• **Mentation**: □BAR   □Confused/   □Drowsy/   □Stuporous   □Coma
               □QAR   Disoriented   Obtunded   (unresponsive
               □Dull   unless aroused by
                                                        noxious stimuli)

• **Skin Elasticity**: □Normal skin turgor, □↓ Skin turgor, □Skin tent, □Gelatinous

• **Mucus Membranes**:
  - *CRT*:_____ [*RI*: 1–2; <1 = compensated shock, sepsis, heat stroke; <2 = acute decompensated shock; >2 = late decompensated shock, decreased cardiac output, hypothermia]
  - *Color*:_____ [*RI*: pink; red = compensated shock, sepsis, heat stroke; pale/white = anemia, shock; blue = cyanosis; yellow = hepatic disease, extravascular hemolysis; brown = met-Hb]
  - *Texture*:_____ [*RI*: moist = hydrated; tacky-to-dry = 5–12% dehydrated]

Physical Exam – Systems Checklist:

- Head:_____ ☐NAF
  - Ears: ☐Debris (mild / mod / sev) (AS / AD / AU),_____ ☐NAF
  - Eyes:_____ ☐NAF
    - Retinal:_____ ☐NAF

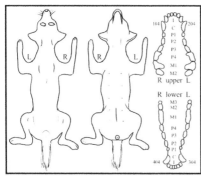 ➝ ⓛ		ⓡ		ⓛ		ⓡ ⬅	
☐	Normal Direct	☐	Normal Indirect	☐	Normal Indirect	☐	Normal Direct
☐	Abnormal Direct	☐	Abnormal Indirect	☐	Abnormal Indirect	☐	Abnormal Direct

- Nose:_____ ☐NAF
  - Oral cavity: ☐Tarter/Gingivitis (mild / mod / sev),_____ ☐NAF
  - Mandibular lnn.: ☐Enlarged Lt., ☐Enlarged Rt.,_____ ☐NAF

- Neck:_____ ☐NAF
  - Superficial cervical lnn.: ☐Enlarged Lt., ☐Enlarged Rt.,_____ ☐NAF
  - Thyroid:_____ ☐NAF

- Thoracic limb:_____ ☐NAF
  - Foot pads:_____ ☐NAF
  - Knuckling:_____ ☐NAF
  - Axillary lnn. [normally absent]:_____ ☐NAF

- Thorax:_____ ☐NAF

- Abdomen:_____ ☐NAF
  - Mammary chain:_____ ☐NAF
  - Penis/ Testicles/ Vulva:_____ ☐NAF
  - Superficial inguinal lnn. [normally absent]:_____ ☐NAF

- Pelvic limb:_____ ☐NAF
  - Foot pads:_____ ☐NAF
  - Knuckling:_____ ☐NAF
  - Popliteal lnn.: ☐Enlarged Lt., ☐Enlarged Rt.,_____ ☐NAF

- Skin:_____ ☐NAF
- Tail:_____ ☐NAF
- Rectal☞☉:_____ ☐NAF

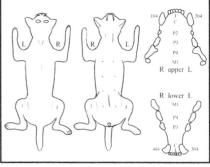

Problems List:

• **Problem #1**:

• **Problem #2**:

• **Problem #3**:

• **Problem #4**:

• **Problem #5**:

Diagnostic Plan	Treatment Plan

Case No._____

Patient	Age	Sex	Breed		Weight
	DOB:	Mn / Mi Fs / Fi	Color:		kg

Owner	Primary Veterinarian	Admit Date/ Time
Name: Phone:	Name: Phone:	Date: Time: AM / PM

• **Presenting Complaint**:_____

_____

• **Medical Hx**:_____

_____

• **When/ where obtained**:   Date:_____ ; ☐Breeder, ☐Shelter, Other:_____

Drug/ Suppl.	Amount	Dose (mg/kg)	Route	Frequency	Date Started

• **Vaccine status – Dog**: ☐Rab ☐Parv ☐Dist ☐Aden; ☐Para ☐Lep ☐Bord ☐Influ ☐Lyme
• **Vaccine status – Cat**: ☐Rab ☐Herp ☐Cali ☐Pan ☐FeLV[kittens]; ☐FIV ☐Chlam ☐Bord
• **Heartworm / Flea & Tick / Intestinal Parasites**:
   ◦ *Last Heartworm Test*: Date:_____, ☐IDK; Test Results: ☐Pos, ☐Neg, ☐IDK
   ◦ *Monthly heartworm preventative*:   ☐no ☐yes, Product:_____
   ◦ *Monthly flea & tick preventative*:   ☐no ☐yes, Product:_____
   ◦ *Monthly dewormer*:   ☐no ☐yes, Product:_____
• **Surgical Hx**:   ☐Spay/Neuter; Date:_____ ; Other:_____
• **Environment**: ☐Indoor, ☐Outdoor, Time spent outdoors/ Other:_____
• **Housemates**: Dogs:_____ Cats:_____ Other:_____
• **Diet**: ☐Wet, ☐Dry; Brand/ Amt.:_____

Appetite	☐Normal, ☐↑, ☐↓
Weight	☐Normal, ☐↑, ☐↓; Past Wt.:_____ kg; Date:_____ ; Δ:_____
Thirst	☐Normal, ☐↑, ☐↓
Urination	☐Normal, ☐↑, ☐↓, ☐Blood, ☐Strain
Defecation	☐Normal, ☐↑, ☐↓, ☐Blood, ☐Strain, ☐Diarrhea, ☐Mucus
Discharge	☐No, ☐Yes; Onset/ Describe:
Cough/ Sneeze	☐No, ☐Yes; Onset/ Describe:
Vomit	☐No, ☐Yes; Onset/ Describe:
Respiration	☐Normal, ☐↑ Rate, ☐↑ Effort
Energy level	☐Normal, ☐Lethargic, ☐Exercise intolerance

• **Travel Hx**: ☐None, Other:_____
• **Exposure to**: ☐Standing water, ☐Wildlife, ☐Board/daycare, ☐Dog park, ☐Groomer
• **Adverse reactions to food/ meds**: ☐None, Other:_____
• **Can give oral meds**: ☐no ☐yes; Helpful Tricks:_____

Physical Exam – General:

- **Body Weight**:_____kg   **Body Condition Score**:_____/9

- **Temperature**:_____°F [*Dog-RI*: 100.9–102.4; *Cat-RI*: 98.1–102.1]

- **Heart**:
  - *Rate*:_____beats/min [Dog-RI: 60–180; Cat-RI: 140–240 (in hospital)]
  - *Rhythm*: ☐Regular, ☐Irregular
  - *Sounds*: ☐None, ☐Split sound, ☐Gallop, ☐Murmur, ☐Muffled
    - *Grade*: ☐1–2[soft, only at PMI], ☐3–4[moderate, mild radiate], ☐5–6[strong radiate, thrill]
    - *Timing*: ☐Systolic, ☐Diastolic, ☐Continuous
    - *PMI*:

	PMI	Over	Anatomic Boundaries
☐	Lt. apex	Mitral valve	5th to 6th ICS at level of CCJ
☐	Lt. base	Ao + Pul outflow	2nd to 4th ICS above the CCJ
☐	Rt. midheart	Tricuspid valve	3rd to 5th ICS near the CCJ
☐	Rt. sternal border	Right ventricle	5th to 7th ICS immediately dorsal to the sternum
☐	Sternal (cat)	Sternum	In cats, PMI offers very little clinical significance.

  - •   *Vertebral Heart Size*: Dog = 8.7–10.5; Cat = 6.9–8.1 (from cranial edge of T4)
  - •   *Innocent Murmur*: Grade 1-2, systolic, left base location, disappear by ~4 months of age, absent clinical signs

- **Pulses**:
  - *Pulse rate*:_____pulses/min
  - *Character*: ☐Sync, ☐Async; ☐Normokinetic, ☐Hyper-, ☐Hypo-, ☐Variable

- **Lungs**:
  - *Respiratory rate*:_____breaths/min [*RI*: 16–30]
  - *Depth/Effort*: ☐Norm, ☐Pant, ☐Deep, ☐Shallow, ☐↑ Insp effort, ☐↑ Exp effort
  - *Sounds/Localization*:
    - ☐Norm BV, ☐Quiet BV, ☐Loud BV, ☐Crack, ☐Wheez, ☐Frict, ☐Muffled
    - ☐All fields, ☐Rt cran, ☐Rt mid, ☐Rt caud, ☐Lt cran, ☐Lt mid, ☐Lt caud
  - *Tracheal Auscultation/ Palpation*: ☐Normal, Other:_____

- **Pain Score**:_____ / 5   Localization:_____

- **Mentation**: ☐BAR   ☐Confused/   ☐Drowsy/   ☐Stuporous   ☐Coma
              ☐QAR   Disoriented   Obtunded   (unresponsive
              ☐Dull   unless aroused by
                                                   noxious stimuli)

- **Skin Elasticity**: ☐Normal skin turgor, ☐↓ Skin turgor, ☐Skin tent, ☐Gelatinous

- **Mucus Membranes**:
  - *CRT*:_____ [*RI*: 1–2; <1 = compensated shock, sepsis, heat stroke; <2 = acute decompensated shock; >2 = late decompensated shock, decreased cardiac output, hypothermia]
  - *Color*:_____ [*RI*: pink; red = compensated shock, sepsis, heat stroke; pale/white = anemia, shock; blue = cyanosis; yellow = hepatic disease, extravascular hemolysis; brown = met-Hb]
  - *Texture*:_____ [*RI*: moist = hydrated; tacky-to-dry = 5–12% dehydrated]

Physical Exam – Systems Checklist:

- Head:_____ ☐NAF
    - Ears: ☐Debris (mild / mod / sev) (AS / AD / AU),_____ ☐NAF
    - Eyes:_____ ☐NAF
        - Retinal:_____ ☐NAF

→⚫L		⚫R		⚫L		⚫R←	
☐	Normal Direct	☐	Normal Indirect	☐	Normal Indirect	☐	Normal Direct
☐	Abnormal Direct	☐	Abnormal Indirect	☐	Abnormal Indirect	☐	Abnormal Direct

- - Nose:_____ ☐NAF
    - Oral cavity: ☐Tarter/Gingivitis (mild / mod / sev),_____ ☐NAF
    - Mandibular lnn.: ☐Enlarged Lt., ☐Enlarged Rt.,_____ ☐NAF

- Neck:_____ ☐NAF
    - Superficial cervical lnn.: ☐Enlarged Lt., ☐Enlarged Rt.,_____ ☐NAF
    - Thyroid:_____ ☐NAF

- Thoracic limb:_____ ☐NAF
    - Foot pads:_____ ☐NAF
    - Knuckling:_____ ☐NAF
    - Axillary lnn. [normally absent]:_____ ☐NAF

- Thorax:_____ ☐NAF

- Abdomen:_____ ☐NAF
    - Mammary chain:_____ ☐NAF
    - Penis/ Testicles/ Vulva:_____ ☐NAF
    - Superficial inguinal lnn. [normally absent]:_____ ☐NAF

- Pelvic limb:_____ ☐NAF
    - Foot pads:_____ ☐NAF
    - Knuckling:_____ ☐NAF
    - Popliteal lnn.: ☐Enlarged Lt., ☐Enlarged Rt.,_____ ☐NAF

- Skin:_____ ☐NAF
- Tail:_____ ☐NAF
- Rectal☞ ☉:_____ ☐NAF

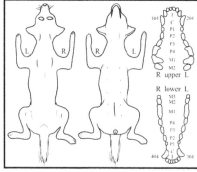

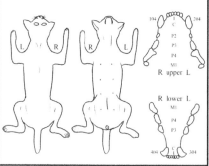

Problems List:

- **Problem #1**:

- **Problem #2**:

- **Problem #3**:

- **Problem #4**:

- **Problem #5**:

Diagnostic Plan	Treatment Plan

Case No._____

Patient	Age	Sex	Breed	Weight
	DOB:	Mn / Mi Fs / Fi	Color:	kg

Owner	Primary Veterinarian	Admit Date/ Time
Name: Phone:	Name: Phone:	Date: Time: AM / PM

• **Presenting Complaint**:_____
_____
_____

• **Medical Hx**:_____
_____
_____

• **When/ where obtained**:   Date:_____; □Breeder, □Shelter, Other:_____

Drug/ Suppl.	Amount	Dose (mg/kg)	Route	Frequency	Date Started

• **Vaccine status – Dog**: □Rab □Parv □Dist □Aden; □Para □Lep □Bord □Influ □Lyme
• **Vaccine status – Cat**: □Rab □Herp □Cali □Pan □FeLV[kittens]; □FIV □Chlam □Bord
• **Heartworm / Flea & Tick / Intestinal Parasites**:
  ◦ *Last Heartworm Test*: Date:_____, □IDK; Test Results: □Pos, □Neg, □IDK
  ◦ *Monthly heartworm preventative*: □no □yes, Product:_____
  ◦ *Monthly flea & tick preventative*: □no □yes, Product:_____
  ◦ *Monthly dewormer*: □no □yes, Product:_____
• **Surgical Hx**: □Spay/Neuter; Date:_____; Other:_____
• **Environment**: □Indoor, □Outdoor, Time spent outdoors/ Other:_____
• **Housemates**: Dogs:_____ Cats:_____ Other:_____
• **Diet**: □Wet, □Dry; Brand/ Amt.:_____

Appetite	□Normal, □↑, □↓
Weight	□Normal, □↑, □↓; Past Wt.:_____ kg; Date:_____; Δ:_____
Thirst	□Normal, □↑, □↓
Urination	□Normal, □↑, □↓, □Blood, □Strain
Defecation	□Normal, □↑, □↓, □Blood, □Strain, □Diarrhea, □Mucus
Discharge	□No, □Yes; Onset/ Describe:
Cough/ Sneeze	□No, □Yes; Onset/ Describe:
Vomit	□No, □Yes; Onset/ Describe:
Respiration	□Normal, □↑ Rate, □↑ Effort
Energy level	□Normal, □Lethargic, □Exercise intolerance

• **Travel Hx**: □None, Other:_____
• **Exposure to**: □Standing water, □Wildlife, □Board/daycare, □Dog park, □Groomer
• **Adverse reactions to food/ meds**: □None, Other:_____
• **Can give oral meds**: □no □yes; Helpful Tricks:_____

Physical Exam – General:

- **Body Weight**:_____kg   **Body Condition Score**:_____/9

- **Temperature**:_____°F [*Dog-RI*: 100.9–102.4; *Cat-RI*: 98.1–102.1]

- **Heart**:
  - *Rate*:_____beats/min [Dog-RI: 60–180; Cat-RI: 140–240 (in hospital)]
  - *Rhythm*: ☐Regular, ☐Irregular
  - *Sounds*: ☐None, ☐Split sound, ☐Gallop, ☐Murmur, ☐Muffled
    - *Grade*: ☐1–2[soft, only at PMI], ☐3–4[moderate, mild radiate], ☐5–6[strong radiate, thrill]
    - *Timing*: ☐Systolic, ☐Diastolic, ☐Continuous
    - *PMI*:

	PMI	Over	Anatomic Boundaries
☐	Lt. apex	Mitral valve	5th to 6th ICS at level of CCJ
☐	Lt. base	Ao + Pul outflow	2nd to 4th ICS above the CCJ
☐	Rt. midheart	Tricuspid valve	3rd to 5th ICS near the CCJ
☐	Rt. sternal border	Right ventricle	5th to 7th ICS immediately dorsal to the sternum
☐	Sternal (cat)	Sternum	In cats, PMI offers very little clinical significance.

   - *Vertebral Heart Size*: Dog = 8.7–10.5; Cat = 6.9–8.1 (from cranial edge of T4)
   - *Innocent Murmur*: Grade 1-2, systolic, left base location, disappear by ~4 months of age, absent clinical signs

- **Pulses**:
  - *Pulse rate*:_____pulses/min
  - *Character*: ☐Sync, ☐Async; ☐Normokinetic, ☐Hyper-, ☐Hypo-, ☐Variable

- **Lungs**:
  - *Respiratory rate*:_____breaths/min [*RI*: 16–30]
  - *Depth/Effort*: ☐Norm, ☐Pant, ☐Deep, ☐Shallow, ☐↑ Insp effort, ☐↑ Exp effort
  - *Sounds/Localization*:
    - ☐Norm BV, ☐Quiet BV, ☐Loud BV, ☐Crack, ☐Wheez, ☐Frict, ☐Muffled
    - ☐All fields, ☐Rt cran, ☐Rt mid, ☐Rt caud, ☐Lt cran, ☐Lt mid, ☐Lt caud
  - *Tracheal Auscultation/ Palpation*: ☐Normal, Other:_____

- **Pain Score**:_____ / 5   Localization:_____

- **Mentation**: ☐BAR   ☐Confused/   ☐Drowsy/   ☐Stuporous   ☐Coma
              ☐QAR   Disoriented   Obtunded   (unresponsive
              ☐Dull   unless aroused by
                                                       noxious stimuli)

- **Skin Elasticity**: ☐Normal skin turgor, ☐↓ Skin turgor, ☐Skin tent, ☐Gelatinous

- **Mucus Membranes**:
  - *CRT*:_____ [*RI*: 1–2; <1 = compensated shock, sepsis, heat stroke; <2 = acute decompensated shock; >2 = late decompensated shock, decreased cardiac output, hypothermia]
  - *Color*:_____ [*RI*: pink; red = compensated shock, sepsis, heat stroke; pale/white = anemia, shock; blue = cyanosis; yellow = hepatic disease, extravascular hemolysis; brown = met-Hb]
  - *Texture*:_____ [*RI*: moist = hydrated; tacky-to-dry = 5–12% dehydrated]

Physical Exam – Systems Checklist:

- Head:_____ ☐NAF
  - Ears: ☐Debris (mild / mod / sev) (AS / AD / AU),_____ ☐NAF
  - Eyes:_____ ☐NAF
    - Retinal:_____ ☐NAF

→ Ⓛ		Ⓡ		Ⓛ		Ⓡ ←	
☐	Normal Direct	☐	Normal Indirect	☐	Normal Indirect	☐	Normal Direct
☐	Abnormal Direct	☐	Abnormal Indirect	☐	Abnormal Indirect	☐	Abnormal Direct

  - Nose:_____ ☐NAF
  - Oral cavity: ☐Tarter/Gingivitis (mild / mod / sev),_____ ☐NAF
  - Mandibular lnn.: ☐Enlarged Lt., ☐Enlarged Rt.,_____ ☐NAF

- Neck:_____ ☐NAF
  - Superficial cervical lnn.: ☐Enlarged Lt., ☐Enlarged Rt.,_____ ☐NAF
  - Thyroid:_____ ☐NAF

- Thoracic limb:_____ ☐NAF
  - Foot pads:_____ ☐NAF
  - Knuckling:_____ ☐NAF
  - Axillary lnn. [normally absent]:_____ ☐NAF

- Thorax:_____ ☐NAF

- Abdomen:_____ ☐NAF
  - Mammary chain:_____ ☐NAF
  - Penis/ Testicles/ Vulva:_____ ☐NAF
  - Superficial inguinal lnn. [normally absent]:_____ ☐NAF

- Pelvic limb:_____ ☐NAF
  - Foot pads:_____ ☐NAF
  - Knuckling:_____ ☐NAF
  - Popliteal lnn.: ☐Enlarged Lt., ☐Enlarged Rt.,_____ ☐NAF

- Skin:_____ ☐NAF
- Tail:_____ ☐NAF
- Rectal☞☉:_____ ☐NAF

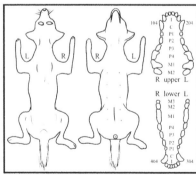
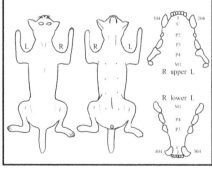

Problems List:

- **Problem #1**:

- **Problem #2**:

- **Problem #3**:

- **Problem #4**:

- **Problem #5**:

Diagnostic Plan	Treatment Plan

Case No._____

Patient	Age	Sex	Breed	Weight
	DOB:	Mn / Mi Fs / Fi	Color:	kg

Owner	Primary Veterinarian	Admit Date/ Time
Name: Phone:	Name: Phone:	Date: Time: AM / PM

• **Presenting Complaint**:_____

_____

• **Medical Hx**:_____

_____

• **When/ where obtained**:   Date:_____ ; □Breeder, □Shelter, Other:_____

Drug/ Suppl.	Amount	Dose (mg/kg)	Route	Frequency	Date Started

• **Vaccine status – Dog**: □Rab □Parv □Dist □Aden; □Para □Lep □Bord □Influ □Lyme
• **Vaccine status – Cat**: □Rab □Herp □Cali □Pan □FeLV[kittens]; □FIV □Chlam □Bord
• **Heartworm / Flea & Tick / Intestinal Parasites**:
  ◦ *Last Heartworm Test*: Date:_____ , □IDK; Test Results: □Pos, □Neg, □IDK
  ◦ *Monthly heartworm preventative*:   □no □yes, Product:_____
  ◦ *Monthly flea & tick preventative*:   □no □yes, Product:_____
  ◦ *Monthly dewormer*:   □no □yes, Product:_____
• **Surgical Hx**: □Spay/Neuter; Date:_____ ; Other:_____
• **Environment**: □Indoor, □Outdoor, Time spent outdoors/ Other:_____
• **Housemates**: Dogs:_____ Cats:_____ Other:_____
• **Diet**: □Wet, □Dry; Brand/ Amt.:_____

Appetite	□Normal, □↑, □↓
Weight	□Normal, □↑, □↓; Past Wt.:_____ kg; Date:_____ ; Δ:_____
Thirst	□Normal, □↑, □↓
Urination	□Normal, □↑, □↓, □Blood, □Strain
Defecation	□Normal, □↑, □↓, □Blood, □Strain, □Diarrhea, □Mucus
Discharge	□No, □Yes; Onset/ Describe:
Cough/ Sneeze	□No, □Yes; Onset/ Describe:
Vomit	□No, □Yes; Onset/ Describe:
Respiration	□Normal, □↑ Rate, □↑ Effort
Energy level	□Normal, □Lethargic, □Exercise intolerance

• **Travel Hx**: □None, Other:_____
• **Exposure to**: □Standing water, □Wildlife, □Board/daycare, □Dog park, □Groomer
• **Adverse reactions to food/ meds**: □None, Other:_____
• **Can give oral meds**: □no □yes; Helpful Tricks:_____

Physical Exam – General:

- **Body Weight**:_____kg   **Body Condition Score**:_____/9

- **Temperature**:_____°F *[Dog-RI: 100.9–102.4; Cat-RI: 98.1–102.1]*

- **Heart**:
  - *Rate*:_____beats/min [Dog-RI: 60–180; Cat-RI: 140–240 (in hospital)]
  - *Rhythm*: ☐Regular, ☐Irregular
  - *Sounds*: ☐None, ☐Split sound, ☐Gallop, ☐Murmur, ☐Muffled
    - *Grade*: ☐1–2[soft, only at PMI], ☐3–4[moderate, mild radiate], ☐5–6[strong radiate, thrill]
    - *Timing*: ☐Systolic, ☐Diastolic, ☐Continuous
    - *PMI*:

	PMI	Over	Anatomic Boundaries
☐	Lt. apex	Mitral valve	5th to 6th ICS at level of CCJ
☐	Lt. base	Ao + Pul outflow	2nd to 4th ICS above the CCJ
☐	Rt. midheart	Tricuspid valve	3rd to 5th ICS near the CCJ
☐	Rt. sternal border	Right ventricle	5th to 7th ICS immediately dorsal to the sternum
☐	Sternal (cat)	Sternum	In cats, PMI offers very little clinical significance.

  - • *Vertebral Heart Size*: Dog = 8.7–10.5; Cat = 6.9–8.1 (from cranial edge of T4)
  - • *Innocent Murmur*: Grade 1-2, systolic, left base location, disappear by ~4 months of age, absent clinical signs

- **Pulses**:
  - *Pulse rate*:_____pulses/min
  - *Character*: ☐Sync, ☐Async; ☐Normokinetic, ☐Hyper-, ☐Hypo-, ☐Variable

- **Lungs**:
  - *Respiratory rate*:_____breaths/min [RI: 16–30]
  - *Depth/Effort*: ☐Norm, ☐Pant, ☐Deep, ☐Shallow, ☐↑ Insp effort, ☐↑ Exp effort
  - *Sounds/Localization*:
    - ☐Norm BV, ☐Quiet BV, ☐Loud BV, ☐Crack, ☐Wheez, ☐Frict, ☐Muffled
    - ☐All fields, ☐Rt cran, ☐Rt mid, ☐Rt caud, ☐Lt cran, ☐Lt mid, ☐Lt caud
  - *Tracheal Auscultation/ Palpation*: ☐Normal, Other:_____

- **Pain Score**:_____ / 5   Localization:_____

- **Mentation**: ☐BAR   ☐Confused/   ☐Drowsy/   ☐Stuporous   ☐Coma
  ☐QAR   Disoriented   Obtunded   (unresponsive
  ☐Dull   unless aroused by
                                              noxious stimuli)

- **Skin Elasticity**: ☐Normal skin turgor, ☐↓ Skin turgor, ☐Skin tent, ☐Gelatinous

- **Mucus Membranes**:
  - *CRT*:_____ [RI: 1–2; <1 = compensated shock, sepsis, heat stroke; <2 = acute decompensated shock; >2 = late decompensated shock, decreased cardiac output, hypothermia]
  - *Color*:_____ [RI: pink; red = compensated shock, sepsis, heat stroke; pale/white = anemia, shock; blue = cyanosis; yellow = hepatic disease, extravascular hemolysis; brown = met-Hb]
  - *Texture*:_____ [RI: moist = hydrated; tacky-to-dry = 5–12% dehydrated]

Physical Exam – Systems Checklist:

- Head:_____ ☐NAF
  - Ears: ☐Debris (mild / mod / sev) (AS / AD / AU),_____ ☐NAF
  - Eyes:_____ ☐NAF
    - Retinal:_____ ☐NAF

➡ Ⓛ	Ⓡ	Ⓛ	Ⓡ ⬅
☐ Normal Direct	☐ Normal Indirect	☐ Normal Indirect	☐ Normal Direct
☐ Abnormal Direct	☐ Abnormal Indirect	☐ Abnormal Indirect	☐ Abnormal Direct

  - Nose:_____ ☐NAF
  - Oral cavity: ☐Tarter/Gingivitis (mild / mod / sev),_____ ☐NAF
  - Mandibular lnn.: ☐Enlarged Lt., ☐Enlarged Rt.,_____ ☐NAF

- Neck:_____ ☐NAF
  - Superficial cervical lnn.: ☐Enlarged Lt., ☐Enlarged Rt.,_____ ☐NAF
  - Thyroid:_____ ☐NAF

- Thoracic limb:_____ ☐NAF
  - Foot pads:_____ ☐NAF
  - Knuckling:_____ ☐NAF
  - Axillary lnn. [normally absent]:_____ ☐NAF

- Thorax:_____ ☐NAF

- Abdomen:_____ ☐NAF
  - Mammary chain:_____ ☐NAF
  - Penis/ Testicles/ Vulva:_____ ☐NAF
  - Superficial inguinal lnn. [normally absent]:_____ ☐NAF

- Pelvic limb:_____ ☐NAF
  - Foot pads:_____ ☐NAF
  - Knuckling:_____ ☐NAF
  - Popliteal lnn.: ☐Enlarged Lt., ☐Enlarged Rt.,_____ ☐NAF

- Skin:_____ ☐NAF
- Tail:_____ ☐NAF
- Rectal☞☉:_____ ☐NAF

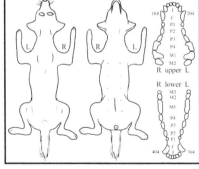
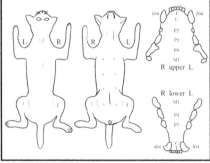

Problems List:

- **Problem #1**:

- **Problem #2**:

- **Problem #3**:

- **Problem #4**:

- **Problem #5**:

Diagnostic Plan	Treatment Plan

Case No._____

Patient	Age	Sex	Breed	Weight
	DOB:	Mn / Mi Fs / Fi	Color:	kg

Owner	Primary Veterinarian	Admit Date/ Time
Name: Phone:	Name: Phone:	Date: Time: AM / PM

• **Presenting Complaint**:_____
_____
_____

• **Medical Hx**:_____
_____
_____

• **When/ where obtained**: Date:_____; ☐Breeder, ☐Shelter, Other:_____

Drug/ Suppl.	Amount	Dose (mg/kg)	Route	Frequency	Date Started

• **Vaccine status – Dog**: ☐Rab ☐Parv ☐Dist ☐Aden; ☐Para ☐Lep ☐Bord ☐Influ ☐Lyme
• **Vaccine status – Cat**: ☐Rab ☐Herp ☐Cali ☐Pan ☐FeLV[kittens]; ☐FIV ☐Chlam ☐Bord
• **Heartworm / Flea & Tick / Intestinal Parasites**:
  ◦ *Last Heartworm Test*: Date:_____, ☐IDK; Test Results: ☐Pos, ☐Neg, ☐IDK
  ◦ *Monthly heartworm preventative*: ☐no ☐yes, Product:_____
  ◦ *Monthly flea & tick preventative*: ☐no ☐yes, Product:_____
  ◦ *Monthly dewormer*: ☐no ☐yes, Product:_____
• **Surgical Hx**: ☐Spay/Neuter; Date:_____; Other:_____
• **Environment**: ☐Indoor, ☐Outdoor, Time spent outdoors/ Other:_____
• **Housemates**: Dogs:_____ Cats:_____ Other:_____
• **Diet**: ☐Wet, ☐Dry; Brand/ Amt.:_____

Appetite	☐Normal, ☐↑, ☐↓
Weight	☐Normal, ☐↑, ☐↓; Past Wt.:_____ kg; Date:_____; Δ:_____
Thirst	☐Normal, ☐↑, ☐↓
Urination	☐Normal, ☐↑, ☐↓, ☐Blood, ☐Strain
Defecation	☐Normal, ☐↑, ☐↓, ☐Blood, ☐Strain, ☐Diarrhea, ☐Mucus
Discharge	☐No, ☐Yes; Onset/ Describe:
Cough/ Sneeze	☐No, ☐Yes; Onset/ Describe:
Vomit	☐No, ☐Yes; Onset/ Describe:
Respiration	☐Normal, ☐↑ Rate, ☐↑ Effort
Energy level	☐Normal, ☐Lethargic, ☐Exercise intolerance

• **Travel Hx**: ☐None, Other:_____
• **Exposure to**: ☐Standing water, ☐Wildlife, ☐Board/daycare, ☐Dog park, ☐Groomer
• **Adverse reactions to food/ meds**: ☐None, Other:_____
• **Can give oral meds**: ☐no ☐yes; Helpful Tricks:_____

Physical Exam – General:

- **Body Weight**:_____kg   **Body Condition Score**:_____/9

- **Temperature**:_____°F [*Dog-RI*: 100.9–102.4; *Cat-RI*: 98.1–102.1]

- **Heart**:
  - *Rate*:_____beats/min [Dog-RI: 60–180; Cat-RI: 140–240 (in hospital)]
  - *Rhythm*: ☐Regular, ☐Irregular
  - *Sounds*: ☐None, ☐Split sound, ☐Gallop, ☐Murmur, ☐Muffled
    - *Grade*: ☐1–2[soft, only at PMI], ☐3–4[moderate, mild radiate], ☐5–6[strong radiate, thrill]
    - *Timing*: ☐Systolic, ☐Diastolic, ☐Continuous
    - *PMI*:

	PMI	Over	Anatomic Boundaries
☐	Lt. apex	Mitral valve	5th to 6th ICS at level of CCJ
☐	Lt. base	Ao + Pul outflow	2nd to 4th ICS above the CCJ
☐	Rt. midheart	Tricuspid valve	3rd to 5th ICS near the CCJ
☐	Rt. sternal border	Right ventricle	5th to 7th ICS immediately dorsal to the sternum
☐	Sternal (cat)	Sternum	In cats, PMI offers very little clinical significance.

  - •   *Vertebral Heart Size*: Dog = 8.7–10.5; Cat = 6.9–8.1 (from cranial edge of T4)
  - •   *Innocent Murmur*: Grade 1-2, systolic, left base location, disappear by ~4 months of age, absent clinical signs

- **Pulses**:
  - *Pulse rate*:_____pulses/min
  - *Character*: ☐Sync, ☐Async; ☐Normokinetic, ☐Hyper-, ☐Hypo-, ☐Variable

- **Lungs**:
  - *Respiratory rate*:_____breaths/min [*RI*: 16–30]
  - *Depth/Effort*: ☐Norm, ☐Pant, ☐Deep, ☐Shallow, ☐↑ Insp effort, ☐↑ Exp effort
  - *Sounds/Localization*:
    - ☐Norm BV, ☐Quiet BV, ☐Loud BV, ☐Crack, ☐Wheez, ☐Frict, ☐Muffled
    - ☐All fields, ☐Rt cran, ☐Rt mid, ☐Rt caud, ☐Lt cran, ☐Lt mid, ☐Lt caud
  - *Tracheal Auscultation/ Palpation*: ☐Normal, Other:_____

- **Pain Score**:_____ / 5   Localization:_____

- **Mentation**: ☐BAR   ☐Confused/   ☐Drowsy/   ☐Stuporous   ☐Coma
  -       ☐QAR   Disoriented   Obtunded   (unresponsive
  -       ☐Dull   unless aroused by
  -   noxious stimuli)

- **Skin Elasticity**: ☐Normal skin turgor, ☐↓ Skin turgor, ☐Skin tent, ☐Gelatinous

- **Mucus Membranes**:
  - *CRT*:_____ [*RI*: 1–2; <1 = compensated shock, sepsis, heat stroke; <2 = acute decompensated shock; >2 = late decompensated shock, decreased cardiac output, hypothermia]
  - *Color*:_____ [*RI*: pink; red = compensated shock, sepsis, heat stroke; pale/white = anemia, shock; blue = cyanosis; yellow = hepatic disease, extravascular hemolysis; brown = met-Hb]
  - *Texture*:_____ [*RI*: moist = hydrated; tacky-to-dry = 5–12% dehydrated]

Physical Exam – Systems Checklist:

- Head:_____ ☐NAF
  - Ears: ☐Debris (mild / mod / sev) (AS / AD / AU),_____ ☐NAF
  - Eyes:_____ ☐NAF
    - Retinal:_____ ☐NAF

→●L		●R		●L		●R←	
☐	Normal Direct	☐	Normal Indirect	☐	Normal Indirect	☐	Normal Direct
☐	Abnormal Direct	☐	Abnormal Indirect	☐	Abnormal Indirect	☐	Abnormal Direct

  - Nose:_____ ☐NAF
  - Oral cavity: ☐Tarter/Gingivitis (mild / mod / sev),_____ ☐NAF
  - Mandibular lnn.: ☐Enlarged Lt., ☐Enlarged Rt.,_____ ☐NAF

- Neck:_____ ☐NAF
  - Superficial cervical lnn.: ☐Enlarged Lt., ☐Enlarged Rt.,_____ ☐NAF
  - Thyroid:_____ ☐NAF

- Thoracic limb:_____ ☐NAF
  - Foot pads:_____ ☐NAF
  - Knuckling:_____ ☐NAF
  - Axillary lnn. [normally absent]:_____ ☐NAF

- Thorax:_____ ☐NAF

- Abdomen:_____ ☐NAF
  - Mammary chain:_____ ☐NAF
  - Penis/ Testicles/ Vulva:_____ ☐NAF
  - Superficial inguinal lnn. [normally absent]:_____ ☐NAF

- Pelvic limb:_____ ☐NAF
  - Foot pads:_____ ☐NAF
  - Knuckling:_____ ☐NAF
  - Popliteal lnn.: ☐Enlarged Lt., ☐Enlarged Rt.,_____ ☐NAF

- Skin:_____ ☐NAF
- Tail:_____ ☐NAF
- Rectal ☞ ☉:_____ ☐NAF

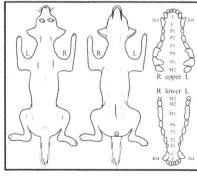

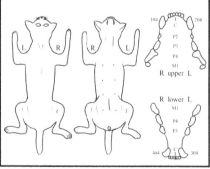

Problems List:

- **Problem #1**:

- **Problem #2**:

- **Problem #3**:

- **Problem #4**:

- **Problem #5**:

Diagnostic Plan	Treatment Plan

Case No._____

Patient	Age	Sex	Breed	Weight
	DOB:	Mn / Mi Fs / Fi	Color:	kg

Owner		Primary Veterinarian	Admit Date/ Time
Name: Phone:		Name: Phone:	Date: Time: AM / PM

• **Presenting Complaint**:_____
_____
_____

• **Medical Hx**:_____
_____
_____

• **When/ where obtained**:   Date:_____; ☐Breeder, ☐Shelter, Other:_____

Drug/ Suppl.	Amount	Dose (mg/kg)	Route	Frequency	Date Started

• **Vaccine status – Dog**: ☐Rab ☐Parv ☐Dist ☐Aden; ☐Para ☐Lep ☐Bord ☐Influ ☐Lyme
• **Vaccine status – Cat**: ☐Rab ☐Herp ☐Cali ☐Pan ☐FeLV[kittens]; ☐FIV ☐Chlam ☐Bord
• **Heartworm / Flea & Tick / Intestinal Parasites**:
  ◦ *Last Heartworm Test*: Date:_____, ☐IDK; Test Results: ☐Pos, ☐Neg, ☐IDK
  ◦ *Monthly heartworm preventative*: ☐no ☐yes, Product:_____
  ◦ *Monthly flea & tick preventative*: ☐no ☐yes, Product:_____
  ◦ *Monthly dewormer*:   ☐no ☐yes, Product:_____
• **Surgical Hx**:   ☐Spay/Neuter; Date:_____; Other:_____
• **Environment**: ☐Indoor, ☐Outdoor, Time spent outdoors/ Other:_____
• **Housemates**: Dogs:_____ Cats:_____ Other:_____
• **Diet**: ☐Wet, ☐Dry; Brand/ Amt.:_____

Appetite	☐Normal, ☐↑, ☐↓
Weight	☐Normal, ☐↑, ☐↓; Past Wt.:_____ kg; Date:_____; Δ:_____
Thirst	☐Normal, ☐↑, ☐↓
Urination	☐Normal, ☐↑, ☐↓, ☐Blood, ☐Strain
Defecation	☐Normal, ☐↑, ☐↓, ☐Blood, ☐Strain, ☐Diarrhea, ☐Mucus
Discharge	☐No, ☐Yes; Onset/ Describe:
Cough/ Sneeze	☐No, ☐Yes; Onset/ Describe:
Vomit	☐No, ☐Yes; Onset/ Describe:
Respiration	☐Normal, ☐↑ Rate, ☐↑ Effort
Energy level	☐Normal, ☐Lethargic, ☐Exercise intolerance

• **Travel Hx**: ☐None, Other:_____
• **Exposure to**: ☐Standing water, ☐Wildlife, ☐Board/daycare, ☐Dog park, ☐Groomer
• **Adverse reactions to food/ meds**: ☐None, Other:_____
• **Can give oral meds**: ☐no ☐yes; Helpful Tricks:_____

Physical Exam – General:

- **Body Weight**:_____kg   **Body Condition Score**:_____/9

- **Temperature**:_____°F [*Dog-RI*: 100.9–102.4; *Cat-RI*: 98.1–102.1]

- **Heart**:
  - *Rate*:_____beats/min [Dog-RI: 60–180; Cat-RI: 140–240 (in hospital)]
  - *Rhythm*:   □Regular, □Irregular
  - *Sounds*:   □None, □Split sound, □Gallop, □Murmur, □Muffled
    - *Grade*:   □1–2[soft, only at PMI], □3–4[moderate, mild radiate], □5–6[strong radiate, thrill]
    - *Timing*: □Systolic, □Diastolic, □Continuous
    - *PMI*:

	PMI	Over	Anatomic Boundaries
□	Lt. apex	Mitral valve	5th to 6th ICS at level of CCJ
□	Lt. base	Ao + Pul outflow	2nd to 4th ICS above the CCJ
□	Rt. midheart	Tricuspid valve	3rd to 5th ICS near the CCJ
□	Rt. sternal border	Right ventricle	5th to 7th ICS immediately dorsal to the sternum
□	Sternal (cat)	Sternum	In cats, PMI offers very little clinical significance.

  - • *Vertebral Heart Size*: Dog = 8.7–10.5; Cat = 6.9–8.1 (from cranial edge of T4)
  - • *Innocent Murmur*: Grade 1-2, systolic, left base location, disappear by ~4 months of age, absent clinical signs

- **Pulses**:
  - *Pulse rate*:_____pulses/min
  - *Character*:   □Sync, □Async; □Normokinetic, □Hyper-, □Hypo-, □Variable

- **Lungs**:
  - *Respiratory rate*:_____breaths/min [*RI*: 16–30]
  - *Depth/Effort*: □Norm, □Pant, □Deep, □Shallow, □↑ Insp effort, □↑ Exp effort
  - *Sounds/Localization*:
    - □Norm BV, □Quiet BV, □Loud BV, □Crack, □Wheez, □Frict, □Muffled
    - □All fields, □Rt cran, □Rt mid, □Rt caud, □Lt cran, □Lt mid, □Lt caud
  - *Tracheal Auscultation/ Palpation*: □Normal, Other:_____

- **Pain Score**:_____ / 5   Localization:_____

- **Mentation**: □BAR   □Confused/   □Drowsy/   □Stuporous   □Coma
                  □QAR   Disoriented   Obtunded   (unresponsive
                  □Dull   unless aroused by
                                                                 noxious stimuli)

- **Skin Elasticity**: □Normal skin turgor, □↓ Skin turgor, □Skin tent, □Gelatinous

- **Mucus Membranes**:
  - *CRT*:_____ [*RI*: 1–2; <1 = compensated shock, sepsis, heat stroke; <2 = acute decompensated shock; >2 = late decompensated shock, decreased cardiac output, hypothermia]
  - *Color*:_____ [*RI*: pink; red = compensated shock, sepsis, heat stroke; pale/white = anemia, shock; blue = cyanosis; yellow = hepatic disease, extravascular hemolysis; brown = met-Hb]
  - *Texture*:_____ [*RI*: moist = hydrated; tacky-to-dry = 5–12% dehydrated]

Physical Exam – Systems Checklist:

- Head:_____ ☐NAF
  - Ears: ☐Debris (mild / mod / sev) (AS / AD / AU),_____ ☐NAF
  - Eyes:_____ ☐NAF
    - Retinal:_____ ☐NAF

→ ⬤L		⬤R		⬤L		⬤R ←	
☐	Normal Direct	☐	Normal Indirect	☐	Normal Indirect	☐	Normal Direct
☐	Abnormal Direct	☐	Abnormal Indirect	☐	Abnormal Indirect	☐	Abnormal Direct

  - Nose:_____ ☐NAF
  - Oral cavity: ☐Tarter/Gingivitis (mild / mod / sev),_____ ☐NAF
  - Mandibular lnn.: ☐Enlarged Lt., ☐Enlarged Rt.,_____ ☐NAF

- Neck:_____ ☐NAF
  - Superficial cervical lnn.: ☐Enlarged Lt., ☐Enlarged Rt.,_____ ☐NAF
  - Thyroid:_____ ☐NAF

- Thoracic limb:_____ ☐NAF
  - Foot pads:_____ ☐NAF
  - Knuckling:_____ ☐NAF
  - Axillary lnn. [normally absent]:_____ ☐NAF

- Thorax:_____ ☐NAF

- Abdomen:_____ ☐NAF
  - Mammary chain:_____ ☐NAF
  - Penis/ Testicles/ Vulva:_____ ☐NAF
  - Superficial inguinal lnn. [normally absent]:_____ ☐NAF

- Pelvic limb:_____ ☐NAF
  - Foot pads:_____ ☐NAF
  - Knuckling:_____ ☐NAF
  - Popliteal lnn.: ☐Enlarged Lt., ☐Enlarged Rt.,_____ ☐NAF

- Skin:_____ ☐NAF
- Tail:_____ ☐NAF
- Rectal☞☉:_____ ☐NAF

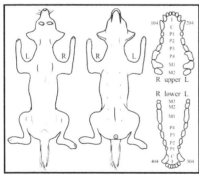
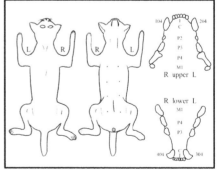

Problems List:

• **Problem #1**:

• **Problem #2**:

• **Problem #3**:

• **Problem #4**:

• **Problem #5**:

Diagnostic Plan	Treatment Plan

Case No._____

Patient	Age	Sex	Breed	Weight
	DOB:	Mn / Mi Fs / Fi	Color:	kg

Owner	Primary Veterinarian	Admit Date/ Time
Name: Phone:	Name: Phone:	Date: Time: AM / PM

• **Presenting Complaint**:_____
_____
_____

• **Medical Hx**:_____
_____
_____

• **When/ where obtained**:   Date:_____ ; ☐Breeder, ☐Shelter, Other:_____

Drug/ Suppl.	Amount	Dose (mg/kg)	Route	Frequency	Date Started

• **Vaccine status – Dog**: ☐Rab ☐Parv ☐Dist ☐Aden; ☐Para ☐Lep ☐Bord ☐Influ ☐Lyme
• **Vaccine status – Cat**: ☐Rab ☐Herp ☐Cali ☐Pan ☐FeLV[kittens]; ☐FIV ☐Chlam ☐Bord
• **Heartworm / Flea & Tick / Intestinal Parasites**:
  ◦ *Last Heartworm Test*: Date:_____, ☐IDK; Test Results: ☐Pos, ☐Neg, ☐IDK
  ◦ *Monthly heartworm preventative*:   ☐no ☐yes, Product:_____
  ◦ *Monthly flea & tick preventative*:   ☐no ☐yes, Product:_____
  ◦ *Monthly dewormer*:   ☐no ☐yes, Product:_____
• **Surgical Hx**:   ☐Spay/Neuter; Date:_____; Other:_____
• **Environment**: ☐Indoor, ☐Outdoor, Time spent outdoors/ Other:_____
• **Housemates**: Dogs:_____ Cats:_____ Other:_____
• **Diet**: ☐Wet, ☐Dry; Brand/ Amt.:_____

Appetite	☐Normal, ☐↑, ☐↓
Weight	☐Normal, ☐↑, ☐↓; Past Wt.:_____ kg; Date:_____; Δ:_____
Thirst	☐Normal, ☐↑, ☐↓
Urination	☐Normal, ☐↑, ☐↓, ☐Blood, ☐Strain
Defecation	☐Normal, ☐↑, ☐↓, ☐Blood, ☐Strain, ☐Diarrhea, ☐Mucus
Discharge	☐No, ☐Yes; Onset/ Describe:
Cough/ Sneeze	☐No, ☐Yes; Onset/ Describe:
Vomit	☐No, ☐Yes; Onset/ Describe:
Respiration	☐Normal, ☐↑ Rate, ☐↑ Effort
Energy level	☐Normal, ☐Lethargic, ☐Exercise intolerance

• **Travel Hx**: ☐None, Other:_____
• **Exposure to**: ☐Standing water, ☐Wildlife, ☐Board/daycare, ☐Dog park, ☐Groomer
• **Adverse reactions to food/ meds**: ☐None, Other:_____
• **Can give oral meds**: ☐no ☐yes; Helpful Tricks:_____

Physical Exam – General:

• **Body Weight**:_____kg   **Body Condition Score**:_____/9

• **Temperature**:_____°F [*Dog-RI*: 100.9–102.4; *Cat-RI*: 98.1–102.1]

• **Heart**:
  ◦ *Rate*:_____beats/min [Dog-RI: 60–180; Cat-RI: 140–240 (in hospital)]
  ◦ *Rhythm*:   ☐Regular, ☐Irregular
  ◦ *Sounds*:   ☐None, ☐Split sound, ☐Gallop, ☐Murmur, ☐Muffled
    ▪ *Grade*: ☐1–2[soft, only at PMI],   ☐3–4[moderate, mild radiate],   ☐5–6[strong radiate, thrill]
    ▪ *Timing*: ☐Systolic, ☐Diastolic, ☐Continuous
    ▪ *PMI*:

	PMI	Over	Anatomic Boundaries
☐	Lt. apex	Mitral valve	5th to 6th ICS at level of CCJ
☐	Lt. base	Ao + Pul outflow	2nd to 4th ICS above the CCJ
☐	Rt. midheart	Tricuspid valve	3rd to 5th ICS near the CCJ
☐	Rt. sternal border	Right ventricle	5th to 7th ICS immediately dorsal to the sternum
☐	Sternal (cat)	Sternum	In cats, PMI offers very little clinical significance.

  • *Vertebral Heart Size*: Dog = 8.7–10.5; Cat = 6.9–8.1 (from cranial edge of T4)
  • *Innocent Murmur*: Grade 1-2, systolic, left base location, disappear by ~4 months of age, absent clinical signs

• **Pulses**:
  ◦ *Pulse rate*:_____pulses/min
  ◦ *Character*:   ☐Sync, ☐Async;   ☐Normokinetic, ☐Hyper-, ☐Hypo-, ☐Variable

• **Lungs**:
  ◦ *Respiratory rate*:_____breaths/min [*RI*: 16–30]
  ◦ *Depth/Effort*: ☐Norm, ☐Pant, ☐Deep, ☐Shallow, ☐↑ Insp effort, ☐↑ Exp effort
  ◦ *Sounds/Localization*:
    ▪ ☐Norm BV, ☐Quiet BV, ☐Loud BV, ☐Crack, ☐Wheez, ☐Frict, ☐Muffled
    ▪ ☐All fields, ☐Rt cran, ☐Rt mid, ☐Rt caud, ☐Lt cran, ☐Lt mid, ☐Lt caud
  ◦ *Tracheal Auscultation/ Palpation*: ☐Normal, Other:_____

• **Pain Score**:_____ / 5   Localization:_____

• **Mentation**: ☐BAR   ☐Confused/   ☐Drowsy/   ☐Stuporous   ☐Coma
                 ☐QAR   Disoriented   Obtunded   (unresponsive
                 ☐Dull   unless aroused by
                                                             noxious stimuli)

• **Skin Elasticity**: ☐Normal skin turgor, ☐↓ Skin turgor, ☐Skin tent, ☐Gelatinous

• **Mucus Membranes**:
  ◦ *CRT*:_____ [*RI*: 1–2; <1 = compensated shock, sepsis, heat stroke; <2 = acute decompensated shock; >2 = late decompensated shock, decreased cardiac output, hypothermia]
  ◦ *Color*:_____ [*RI*: pink; red = compensated shock, sepsis, heat stroke; pale/white = anemia, shock; blue = cyanosis; yellow = hepatic disease, extravascular hemolysis; brown = met-Hb]
  ◦ *Texture*:_____ [*RI*: moist = hydrated; tacky-to-dry = 5–12% dehydrated]

Physical Exam – Systems Checklist:

- Head: _____ ☐NAF
  - Ears: ☐Debris (mild / mod / sev) (AS / AD / AU), _____ ☐NAF
  - Eyes: _____ ☐NAF
    - Retinal: _____ ☐NAF

	➔ Ⓛ		Ⓡ		Ⓛ		Ⓡ ⬅
☐	Normal Direct	☐	Normal Indirect	☐	Normal Indirect	☐	Normal Direct
☐	Abnormal Direct	☐	Abnormal Indirect	☐	Abnormal Indirect	☐	Abnormal Direct

  - Nose: _____ ☐NAF
  - Oral cavity: ☐Tarter/Gingivitis (mild / mod / sev), _____ ☐NAF
  - Mandibular lnn.: ☐Enlarged Lt., ☐Enlarged Rt., _____ ☐NAF

- Neck: _____ ☐NAF
  - Superficial cervical lnn.: ☐Enlarged Lt., ☐Enlarged Rt., ____ ☐NAF
  - Thyroid: _____ ☐NAF

- Thoracic limb: _____ ☐NAF
  - Foot pads: _____ ☐NAF
  - Knuckling: _____ ☐NAF
  - Axillary lnn. [normally absent]: _____ ☐NAF

- Thorax: _____ ☐NAF

- Abdomen: _____ ☐NAF
  - Mammary chain: _____ ☐NAF
  - Penis/ Testicles/ Vulva: _____ ☐NAF
  - Superficial inguinal lnn. [normally absent]: _____ ☐NAF

- Pelvic limb: _____ ☐NAF
  - Foot pads: _____ ☐NAF
  - Knuckling: _____ ☐NAF
  - Popliteal lnn.: ☐Enlarged Lt., ☐Enlarged Rt., _____ ☐NAF

- Skin: _____ ☐NAF
- Tail: _____ ☐NAF
- Rectal☞⊙: _____ ☐NAF

Problems List:

• **Problem #1**:

• **Problem #2**:

• **Problem #3**:

• **Problem #4**:

• **Problem #5**:

Diagnostic Plan	Treatment Plan

Case No._____

Patient	Age	Sex	Breed	Weight
	DOB:	Mn / Mi Fs / Fi	Color:	kg

Owner	Primary Veterinarian	Admit Date/ Time
Name: Phone:	Name: Phone:	Date: Time: AM / PM

• **Presenting Complaint**:_____
_____
_____

• **Medical Hx**:_____
_____
_____

• **When/ where obtained**:   Date:_____; ☐Breeder, ☐Shelter, Other:_____

Drug/ Suppl.	Amount	Dose (mg/kg)	Route	Frequency	Date Started

• **Vaccine status – Dog**: ☐Rab ☐Parv ☐Dist ☐Aden; ☐Para ☐Lep ☐Bord ☐Influ ☐Lyme
• **Vaccine status – Cat**: ☐Rab ☐Herp ☐Cali ☐Pan ☐FeLV[kittens]; ☐FIV ☐Chlam ☐Bord
• **Heartworm / Flea & Tick / Intestinal Parasites**:
   ◦ *Last Heartworm Test*: Date:_____, ☐IDK; Test Results: ☐Pos, ☐Neg, ☐IDK
   ◦ *Monthly heartworm preventative*:   ☐no ☐yes, Product:_____
   ◦ *Monthly flea & tick preventative*:   ☐no ☐yes, Product:_____
   ◦ *Monthly dewormer*:   ☐no ☐yes, Product:_____
• **Surgical Hx**:   ☐Spay/Neuter; Date:_____; Other:_____
• **Environment**: ☐Indoor, ☐Outdoor, Time spent outdoors/ Other:_____
• **Housemates**: Dogs:_____ Cats:_____ Other:_____
• **Diet**: ☐Wet, ☐Dry; Brand/ Amt.:_____

Appetite	☐Normal, ☐↑, ☐↓
Weight	☐Normal, ☐↑, ☐↓; Past Wt.:_____ kg; Date:_____; Δ:_____
Thirst	☐Normal, ☐↑, ☐↓
Urination	☐Normal, ☐↑, ☐↓, ☐Blood, ☐Strain
Defecation	☐Normal, ☐↑, ☐↓, ☐Blood, ☐Strain, ☐Diarrhea, ☐Mucus
Discharge	☐No, ☐Yes; Onset/ Describe:
Cough/ Sneeze	☐No, ☐Yes; Onset/ Describe:
Vomit	☐No, ☐Yes; Onset/ Describe:
Respiration	☐Normal, ☐↑ Rate, ☐↑ Effort
Energy level	☐Normal, ☐Lethargic, ☐Exercise intolerance

• **Travel Hx**: ☐None, Other:_____
• **Exposure to**: ☐Standing water, ☐Wildlife, ☐Board/daycare, ☐Dog park, ☐Groomer
• **Adverse reactions to food/ meds**: ☐None, Other:_____
• **Can give oral meds**: ☐no ☐yes; Helpful Tricks:_____

Physical Exam – General:

- **Body Weight**:_____kg   **Body Condition Score**:_____/9

- **Temperature**:_____°F [*Dog-RI*: 100.9–102.4; *Cat-RI*: 98.1–102.1]

- **Heart**:
    - *Rate*:_____beats/min [Dog-RI: 60–180; Cat-RI: 140–240 (in hospital)]
    - *Rhythm*:   □Regular, □Irregular
    - *Sounds*:   □None, □Split sound, □Gallop, □Murmur, □Muffled
        - *Grade*:   □1–2[soft, only at PMI],   □3–4[moderate, mild radiate],   □5–6[strong radiate, thrill]
        - *Timing*: □Systolic, □Diastolic, □Continuous
        - *PMI*:

	PMI	Over	Anatomic Boundaries
□	Lt. apex	Mitral valve	5th to 6th ICS at level of CCJ
□	Lt. base	Ao + Pul outflow	2nd to 4th ICS above the CCJ
□	Rt. midheart	Tricuspid valve	3rd to 5th ICS near the CCJ
□	Rt. sternal border	Right ventricle	5th to 7th ICS immediately dorsal to the sternum
□	Sternal (cat)	Sternum	In cats, PMI offers very little clinical significance.

- •   *Vertebral Heart Size*: Dog = 8.7–10.5; Cat = 6.9–8.1 (from cranial edge of T4)
- •   *Innocent Murmur*: Grade 1-2, systolic, left base location, disappear by ~4 months of age, absent clinical signs

- **Pulses**:
    - *Pulse rate*:_____pulses/min
    - *Character*:   □Sync, □Async;   □Normokinetic, □Hyper-, □Hypo-, □Variable

- **Lungs**:
    - *Respiratory rate*:_____breaths/min [*RI*: 16–30]
    - *Depth/Effort*: □Norm, □Pant, □Deep, □Shallow, □↑ Insp effort, □↑ Exp effort
    - *Sounds/Localization*:
        - □Norm BV, □Quiet BV, □Loud BV, □Crack, □Wheez, □Frict, □Muffled
        - □All fields, □Rt cran, □Rt mid, □Rt caud, □Lt cran, □Lt mid, □Lt caud
    - *Tracheal Auscultation/ Palpation*: □Normal, Other:_____

- **Pain Score**:_____ / 5   Localization:_____

- **Mentation**: □BAR   □Confused/   □Drowsy/   □Stuporous   □Coma
                 □QAR   Disoriented   Obtunded   (unresponsive
                 □Dull   unless aroused by
                                                                     noxious stimuli)

- **Skin Elasticity**: □Normal skin turgor, □↓ Skin turgor, □Skin tent, □Gelatinous

- **Mucus Membranes**:
    - *CRT*:_____ [*RI*: 1–2; <1 = compensated shock, sepsis, heat stroke; <2 = acute decompensated shock; >2 = late decompensated shock, decreased cardiac output, hypothermia]
    - *Color*:_____ [*RI*: pink; red = compensated shock, sepsis, heat stroke; pale/white = anemia, shock; blue = cyanosis; yellow = hepatic disease, extravascular hemolysis; brown = met-Hb]
    - *Texture*:_____ [*RI*: moist = hydrated; tacky-to-dry = 5–12% dehydrated]

Physical Exam – Systems Checklist:

- Head:_____ ☐NAF
  - Ears: ☐Debris (mild / mod / sev) (AS / AD / AU),_____ ☐NAF
  - Eyes:_____ ☐NAF
    - Retinal:_____ ☐NAF

→ Ⓛ		Ⓡ		Ⓛ		Ⓡ ←	
☐	Normal Direct	☐	Normal Indirect	☐	Normal Indirect	☐	Normal Direct
☐	Abnormal Direct	☐	Abnormal Indirect	☐	Abnormal Indirect	☐	Abnormal Direct

  - Nose:_____ ☐NAF
  - Oral cavity: ☐Tarter/Gingivitis (mild / mod / sev),_____ ☐NAF
  - Mandibular lnn.: ☐Enlarged Lt., ☐Enlarged Rt.,_____ ☐NAF

- Neck:_____ ☐NAF
  - Superficial cervical lnn.: ☐Enlarged Lt., ☐Enlarged Rt.,_____ ☐NAF
  - Thyroid:_____ ☐NAF

- Thoracic limb:_____ ☐NAF
  - Foot pads:_____ ☐NAF
  - Knuckling:_____ ☐NAF
  - Axillary lnn. [normally absent]:_____ ☐NAF

- Thorax:_____ ☐NAF

- Abdomen:_____ ☐NAF
  - Mammary chain:_____ ☐NAF
  - Penis/ Testicles/ Vulva:_____ ☐NAF
  - Superficial inguinal lnn. [normally absent]:_____ ☐NAF

- Pelvic limb:_____ ☐NAF
  - Foot pads:_____ ☐NAF
  - Knuckling:_____ ☐NAF
  - Popliteal lnn.: ☐Enlarged Lt., ☐Enlarged Rt.,_____ ☐NAF

- Skin:_____ ☐NAF
- Tail:_____ ☐NAF
- Rectal☞ ☉:_____ ☐NAF

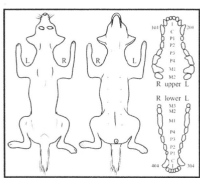

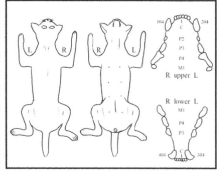

Problems List:

• **Problem #1**:

• **Problem #2**:

• **Problem #3**:

• **Problem #4**:

• **Problem #5**:

Diagnostic Plan	Treatment Plan

Case No._____

Patient		Age	Sex	Breed	Weight
	DOB:		Mn / Mi Fs / Fi	Color:	kg

Owner		Primary Veterinarian	Admit Date/ Time
Name: Phone:		Name: Phone:	Date: Time: AM / PM

• **Presenting Complaint**:_____
_____
_____

• **Medical Hx**:_____
_____
_____

• **When/ where obtained**:   Date:_____ ;   ☐Breeder, ☐Shelter, Other:_____

Drug/ Suppl.	Amount	Dose (mg/kg)	Route	Frequency	Date Started

• **Vaccine status – Dog**: ☐Rab ☐Parv ☐Dist ☐Aden; ☐Para ☐Lep ☐Bord ☐Influ ☐Lyme
• **Vaccine status – Cat**: ☐Rab ☐Herp ☐Cali ☐Pan ☐FeLV[kittens]; ☐FIV ☐Chlam ☐Bord
• **Heartworm / Flea & Tick / Intestinal Parasites**:
  ◦ *Last Heartworm Test*: Date:_____, ☐IDK; Test Results: ☐Pos, ☐Neg, ☐IDK
  ◦ *Monthly heartworm preventative*:   ☐no ☐yes,   Product:_____
  ◦ *Monthly flea & tick preventative*:   ☐no ☐yes,   Product:_____
  ◦ *Monthly dewormer*:   ☐no ☐yes,   Product:_____
• **Surgical Hx**:   ☐Spay/Neuter; Date:_____;   Other:_____
• **Environment**: ☐Indoor, ☐Outdoor, Time spent outdoors/ Other:_____
• **Housemates**: Dogs:_____ Cats:_____ Other:_____
• **Diet**: ☐Wet, ☐Dry; Brand/ Amt.:_____

Appetite	☐Normal, ☐↑, ☐↓
Weight	☐Normal, ☐↑, ☐↓; Past Wt.:_____ kg; Date:_____ ; Δ:_____
Thirst	☐Normal, ☐↑, ☐↓
Urination	☐Normal, ☐↑, ☐↓, ☐Blood, ☐Strain
Defecation	☐Normal, ☐↑, ☐↓, ☐Blood, ☐Strain, ☐Diarrhea, ☐Mucus
Discharge	☐No, ☐Yes; Onset/ Describe:
Cough/ Sneeze	☐No, ☐Yes; Onset/ Describe:
Vomit	☐No, ☐Yes; Onset/ Describe:
Respiration	☐Normal, ☐↑ Rate, ☐↑ Effort
Energy level	☐Normal, ☐Lethargic, ☐Exercise intolerance

• **Travel Hx**: ☐None, Other:_____
• **Exposure to**: ☐Standing water, ☐Wildlife, ☐Board/daycare, ☐Dog park, ☐Groomer
• **Adverse reactions to food/ meds**: ☐None, Other:_____
• **Can give oral meds**: ☐no ☐yes; Helpful Tricks:_____

Physical Exam – General:

- **Body Weight**:_____kg   **Body Condition Score**:_____/9

- **Temperature**:_____°F [*Dog-RI*: 100.9–102.4;   *Cat-RI*: 98.1–102.1]

- **Heart**:
  - *Rate*:_____beats/min [Dog-RI: 60–180;   Cat-RI: 140–240 (in hospital)]
  - *Rhythm*:   ☐Regular, ☐Irregular
  - *Sounds*:   ☐None, ☐Split sound, ☐Gallop, ☐Murmur, ☐Muffled
    - *Grade*:   ☐1–2[soft, only at PMI],   ☐3–4[moderate, mild radiate],   ☐5–6[strong radiate, thrill]
    - *Timing*: ☐Systolic, ☐Diastolic, ☐Continuous
    - *PMI*:

	PMI	Over	Anatomic Boundaries
☐	Lt. apex	Mitral valve	5th to 6th ICS at level of CCJ
☐	Lt. base	Ao + Pul outflow	2nd to 4th ICS above the CCJ
☐	Rt. midheart	Tricuspid valve	3rd to 5th ICS near the CCJ
☐	Rt. sternal border	Right ventricle	5th to 7th ICS immediately dorsal to the sternum
☐	Sternal (cat)	Sternum	In cats, PMI offers very little clinical significance.

  - • *Vertebral Heart Size*: Dog = 8.7–10.5; Cat = 6.9–8.1 (from cranial edge of T4)
  - • *Innocent Murmur*: Grade 1-2, systolic, left base location, disappear by ~4 months of age, absent clinical signs

- **Pulses**:
  - *Pulse rate*:_____pulses/min
  - *Character*:   ☐Sync, ☐Async;   ☐Normokinetic, ☐Hyper-, ☐Hypo-, ☐Variable

- **Lungs**:
  - *Respiratory rate*:_____breaths/min [*RI*: 16–30]
  - *Depth/Effort*: ☐Norm, ☐Pant, ☐Deep, ☐Shallow, ☐↑ Insp effort, ☐↑ Exp effort
  - *Sounds/Localization*:
    - ☐Norm BV, ☐Quiet BV, ☐Loud BV, ☐Crack, ☐Wheez, ☐Frict, ☐Muffled
    - ☐All fields, ☐Rt cran, ☐Rt mid, ☐Rt caud, ☐Lt cran, ☐Lt mid, ☐Lt caud
  - *Tracheal Auscultation/ Palpation*: ☐Normal, Other:_____

- **Pain Score**:_____ / 5   Localization:_____

- **Mentation**: ☐BAR   ☐Confused/   ☐Drowsy/   ☐Stuporous   ☐Coma
             ☐QAR   Disoriented   Obtunded   (unresponsive
             ☐Dull   unless aroused by
                                                             noxious stimuli)

- **Skin Elasticity**: ☐Normal skin turgor, ☐↓ Skin turgor, ☐Skin tent, ☐Gelatinous

- **Mucus Membranes**:
  - *CRT*:_____ [*RI*: 1–2; <1 = compensated shock, sepsis, heat stroke; <2 = acute decompensated shock; >2 = late decompensated shock, decreased cardiac output, hypothermia]
  - *Color*:_____ [*RI*: pink; red = compensated shock, sepsis, heat stroke; pale/white = anemia, shock; blue = cyanosis; yellow = hepatic disease, extravascular hemolysis; brown = met-Hb]
  - *Texture*:_____ [*RI*: moist = hydrated; tacky-to-dry = 5–12% dehydrated]

<u>Physical Exam – Systems Checklist</u>:

- Head:_____ □NAF
  - ○ Ears: □Debris (mild / mod / sev) (AS / AD / AU),_____ □NAF
  - ○ Eyes:_____ □NAF
    - ▪ Retinal:_____ □NAF

→ Ⓛ		Ⓡ		Ⓛ		Ⓡ ←	
□	Normal Direct	□	Normal Indirect	□	Normal Indirect	□	Normal Direct
□	Abnormal Direct	□	Abnormal Indirect	□	Abnormal Indirect	□	Abnormal Direct

  - ○ Nose:_____ □NAF
  - ○ Oral cavity: □Tarter/Gingivitis (mild / mod / sev),_____ □NAF
  - ○ Mandibular lnn.: □Enlarged Lt., □Enlarged Rt.,_____ □NAF

- Neck:_____ □NAF
  - ○ Superficial cervical lnn.: □Enlarged Lt., □Enlarged Rt.,_____ □NAF
  - ○ Thyroid:_____ □NAF

- Thoracic limb:_____ □NAF
  - ○ Foot pads:_____ □NAF
  - ○ Knuckling:_____ □NAF
  - ○ Axillary lnn. [normally absent]:_____ □NAF

- Thorax:_____ □NAF

- Abdomen:_____ □NAF
  - ○ Mammary chain:_____ □NAF
  - ○ Penis/ Testicles/ Vulva:_____ □NAF
  - ○ Superficial inguinal lnn. [normally absent]:_____ □NAF

- Pelvic limb:_____ □NAF
  - ○ Foot pads:_____ □NAF
  - ○ Knuckling:_____ □NAF
  - ○ Popliteal lnn.: □Enlarged Lt., □Enlarged Rt.,_____ □NAF

- Skin:_____ □NAF
- Tail:_____ □NAF
- Rectal☞☉:_____ □NAF

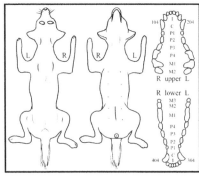

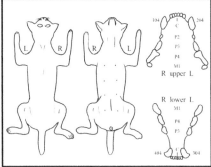

Problems List:

• **Problem #1**:

• **Problem #2**:

• **Problem #3**:

• **Problem #4**:

• **Problem #5**:

Diagnostic Plan	Treatment Plan

Case No._____

Patient	Age	Sex	Breed	Weight
	DOB:	Mn / Mi Fs / Fi	Color:	kg

Owner	Primary Veterinarian	Admit Date/ Time
Name: Phone:	Name: Phone:	Date: Time: AM / PM

• **Presenting Complaint**:_____

_____

• **Medical Hx**:_____

_____

• **When/ where obtained**:   Date:_____ ; □Breeder, □Shelter, Other:_____

Drug/ Suppl.	Amount	Dose (mg/kg)	Route	Frequency	Date Started

• **Vaccine status – Dog**: □Rab □Parv □Dist □Aden; □Para □Lep □Bord □Influ □Lyme
• **Vaccine status – Cat**: □Rab □Herp □Cali □Pan □FeLV[kittens]; □FIV □Chlam □Bord
• **Heartworm / Flea & Tick / Intestinal Parasites**:
  ◦ *Last Heartworm Test*: Date:_____ , □IDK; Test Results: □Pos, □Neg, □IDK
  ◦ *Monthly heartworm preventative*:   □no □yes, Product:_____
  ◦ *Monthly flea & tick preventative*:   □no □yes, Product:_____
  ◦ *Monthly dewormer*:   □no □yes, Product:_____
• **Surgical Hx**: □Spay/Neuter; Date:_____ ; Other:_____
• **Environment**: □Indoor, □Outdoor, Time spent outdoors/ Other:_____
• **Housemates**: Dogs:_____ Cats:_____ Other:_____
• **Diet**: □Wet, □Dry; Brand/ Amt.:_____

Appetite	□Normal, □↑, □↓
Weight	□Normal, □↑, □↓; Past Wt.:_____ kg; Date:_____ ; Δ:_____
Thirst	□Normal, □↑, □↓
Urination	□Normal, □↑, □↓, □Blood, □Strain
Defecation	□Normal, □↑, □↓, □Blood, □Strain, □Diarrhea, □Mucus
Discharge	□No, □Yes; Onset/ Describe:
Cough/ Sneeze	□No, □Yes; Onset/ Describe:
Vomit	□No, □Yes; Onset/ Describe:
Respiration	□Normal, □↑ Rate, □↑ Effort
Energy level	□Normal, □Lethargic, □Exercise intolerance

• **Travel Hx**: □None, Other:_____
• **Exposure to**: □Standing water, □Wildlife, □Board/daycare, □Dog park, □Groomer
• **Adverse reactions to food/ meds**: □None, Other:_____
• **Can give oral meds**: □no □yes; Helpful Tricks:_____

Physical Exam – General:

- **Body Weight**:_____kg   **Body Condition Score**:_____/9

- **Temperature**:_____°F [*Dog-RI*: 100.9–102.4; *Cat-RI*: 98.1–102.1]

- **Heart**:
  - *Rate*:_____beats/min [Dog-RI: 60–180; Cat-RI: 140–240 (in hospital)]
  - *Rhythm*: ☐Regular, ☐Irregular
  - *Sounds*: ☐None, ☐Split sound, ☐Gallop, ☐Murmur, ☐Muffled
    - *Grade*: ☐1–2[soft, only at PMI], ☐3–4[moderate, mild radiate], ☐5–6[strong radiate, thrill]
    - *Timing*: ☐Systolic, ☐Diastolic, ☐Continuous
    - *PMI*:

	PMI	Over	Anatomic Boundaries
☐	Lt. apex	Mitral valve	5th to 6th ICS at level of CCJ
☐	Lt. base	Ao + Pul outflow	2nd to 4th ICS above the CCJ
☐	Rt. midheart	Tricuspid valve	3rd to 5th ICS near the CCJ
☐	Rt. sternal border	Right ventricle	5th to 7th ICS immediately dorsal to the sternum
☐	Sternal (cat)	Sternum	In cats, PMI offers very little clinical significance.

- • *Vertebral Heart Size*: Dog = 8.7–10.5; Cat = 6.9–8.1 (from cranial edge of T4)
- • *Innocent Murmur*: Grade 1-2, systolic, left base location, disappear by ~4 months of age, absent clinical signs

- **Pulses**:
  - *Pulse rate*:_____pulses/min
  - *Character*: ☐Sync, ☐Async; ☐Normokinetic, ☐Hyper-, ☐Hypo-, ☐Variable

- **Lungs**:
  - *Respiratory rate*:_____breaths/min [*RI*: 16–30]
  - *Depth/Effort*: ☐Norm, ☐Pant, ☐Deep, ☐Shallow, ☐↑ Insp effort, ☐↑ Exp effort
  - *Sounds/Localization*:
    - ☐Norm BV, ☐Quiet BV, ☐Loud BV, ☐Crack, ☐Wheez, ☐Frict, ☐Muffled
    - ☐All fields, ☐Rt cran, ☐Rt mid, ☐Rt caud, ☐Lt cran, ☐Lt mid, ☐Lt caud
  - *Tracheal Auscultation/ Palpation*: ☐Normal, Other:_____

- **Pain Score**:_____ / 5   Localization:_____

- **Mentation**: ☐BAR   ☐Confused/   ☐Drowsy/   ☐Stuporous   ☐Coma
          ☐QAR   Disoriented   Obtunded   (unresponsive
          ☐Dull   unless aroused by
                                                 noxious stimuli)

- **Skin Elasticity**: ☐Normal skin turgor, ☐↓ Skin turgor, ☐Skin tent, ☐Gelatinous

- **Mucus Membranes**:
  - *CRT*:_____ [*RI*: 1–2; <1 = compensated shock, sepsis, heat stroke; <2 = acute decompensated shock; >2 = late decompensated shock, decreased cardiac output, hypothermia]
  - *Color*:_____ [*RI*: pink; red = compensated shock, sepsis, heat stroke; pale/white = anemia, shock; blue = cyanosis; yellow = hepatic disease, extravascular hemolysis; brown = met-Hb]
  - *Texture*:_____ [*RI*: moist = hydrated; tacky-to-dry = 5–12% dehydrated]

Physical Exam – Systems Checklist:

- Head: _____ ☐NAF
  - Ears: ☐Debris (mild / mod / sev) (AS / AD / AU), _____ ☐NAF
  - Eyes: _____ ☐NAF
    - Retinal: _____ ☐NAF

	→ 🔵 L		🔴 R		🔵 L		🔴 R ←
☐	Normal Direct	☐	Normal Indirect	☐	Normal Indirect	☐	Normal Direct
☐	Abnormal Direct	☐	Abnormal Indirect	☐	Abnormal Indirect	☐	Abnormal Direct

  - Nose: _____ ☐NAF
  - Oral cavity: ☐Tarter/Gingivitis (mild / mod / sev), _____ ☐NAF
  - Mandibular lnn.: ☐Enlarged Lt., ☐Enlarged Rt., _____ ☐NAF

- Neck: _____ ☐NAF
  - Superficial cervical lnn.: ☐Enlarged Lt., ☐Enlarged Rt., _____ ☐NAF
  - Thyroid: _____ ☐NAF

- Thoracic limb: _____ ☐NAF
  - Foot pads: _____ ☐NAF
  - Knuckling: _____ ☐NAF
  - Axillary lnn. [normally absent]: _____ ☐NAF

- Thorax: _____ ☐NAF

- Abdomen: _____ ☐NAF
  - Mammary chain: _____ ☐NAF
  - Penis/ Testicles/ Vulva: _____ ☐NAF
  - Superficial inguinal lnn. [normally absent]: _____ ☐NAF

- Pelvic limb: _____ ☐NAF
  - Foot pads: _____ ☐NAF
  - Knuckling: _____ ☐NAF
  - Popliteal lnn.: ☐Enlarged Lt., ☐Enlarged Rt., _____ ☐NAF

- Skin: _____ ☐NAF
- Tail: _____ ☐NAF
- Rectal☞☉: _____ ☐NAF

Problems List:

• **Problem #1**:

• **Problem #2**:

• **Problem #3**:

• **Problem #4**:

• **Problem #5**:

Diagnostic Plan	Treatment Plan

Case No._____

Patient	Age	Sex	Breed	Weight
	DOB:	Mn / Mi Fs / Fi	Color:	kg

Owner	Primary Veterinarian	Admit Date/ Time
Name: Phone:	Name: Phone:	Date: Time: AM / PM

• **Presenting Complaint**:_____
_____
_____

• **Medical Hx**:_____
_____
_____

• **When/ where obtained**:   Date:_____; □Breeder, □Shelter, Other:_____

Drug/ Suppl.	Amount	Dose (mg/kg)	Route	Frequency	Date Started

• **Vaccine status – Dog**: □Rab □Parv □Dist □Aden; □Para □Lep □Bord □Influ □Lyme
• **Vaccine status – Cat**: □Rab □Herp □Cali □Pan □FeLV[kittens]; □FIV □Chlam □Bord
• **Heartworm / Flea & Tick / Intestinal Parasites**:
   ◦ *Last Heartworm Test*: Date:_____, □IDK; Test Results: □Pos, □Neg, □IDK
   ◦ *Monthly heartworm preventative*:   □no □yes, Product:_____
   ◦ *Monthly flea & tick preventative*:   □no □yes, Product:_____
   ◦ *Monthly dewormer*:   □no □yes, Product:_____
• **Surgical Hx**: □Spay/Neuter; Date:_____; Other:_____
• **Environment**: □Indoor, □Outdoor, Time spent outdoors/ Other:_____
• **Housemates**: Dogs:_____ Cats:_____ Other:_____
• **Diet**: □Wet, □Dry; Brand/ Amt.:_____

Appetite	□Normal, □↑, □↓
Weight	□Normal, □↑, □↓; Past Wt.:_____ kg; Date:_____; Δ:_____
Thirst	□Normal, □↑, □↓
Urination	□Normal, □↑, □↓, □Blood, □Strain
Defecation	□Normal, □↑, □↓, □Blood, □Strain, □Diarrhea, □Mucus
Discharge	□No, □Yes; Onset/ Describe:
Cough/ Sneeze	□No, □Yes; Onset/ Describe:
Vomit	□No, □Yes; Onset/ Describe:
Respiration	□Normal, □↑ Rate, □↑ Effort
Energy level	□Normal, □Lethargic, □Exercise intolerance

• **Travel Hx**: □None, Other:_____
• **Exposure to**: □Standing water, □Wildlife, □Board/daycare, □Dog park, □Groomer
• **Adverse reactions to food/ meds**: □None, Other:_____
• **Can give oral meds**: □no □yes; Helpful Tricks:_____

Physical Exam – General:

- **Body Weight**:_____kg   **Body Condition Score**:_____/9

- **Temperature**:_____°F [*Dog-RI*: 100.9–102.4; *Cat-RI*: 98.1–102.1]

- **Heart**:
  - *Rate*:_____beats/min [Dog-RI: 60–180; Cat-RI: 140–240 (in hospital)]
  - *Rhythm*: ☐Regular, ☐Irregular
  - *Sounds*: ☐None, ☐Split sound, ☐Gallop, ☐Murmur, ☐Muffled
    - *Grade*: ☐1–2[soft, only at PMI], ☐3–4[moderate, mild radiate], ☐5–6[strong radiate, thrill]
    - *Timing*: ☐Systolic, ☐Diastolic, ☐Continuous
    - *PMI*:

	PMI	Over	Anatomic Boundaries
☐	Lt. apex	Mitral valve	5th to 6th ICS at level of CCJ
☐	Lt. base	Ao + Pul outflow	2nd to 4th ICS above the CCJ
☐	Rt. midheart	Tricuspid valve	3rd to 5th ICS near the CCJ
☐	Rt. sternal border	Right ventricle	5th to 7th ICS immediately dorsal to the sternum
☐	Sternal (cat)	Sternum	In cats, PMI offers very little clinical significance.

  - • *Vertebral Heart Size*: Dog = 8.7–10.5; Cat = 6.9–8.1 (from cranial edge of T4)
  - • *Innocent Murmur*: Grade 1-2, systolic, left base location, disappear by ~4 months of age, absent clinical signs

- **Pulses**:
  - *Pulse rate*:_____pulses/min
  - *Character*: ☐Sync, ☐Async; ☐Normokinetic, ☐Hyper-, ☐Hypo-, ☐Variable

- **Lungs**:
  - *Respiratory rate*:_____breaths/min [*RI*: 16–30]
  - *Depth/Effort*: ☐Norm, ☐Pant, ☐Deep, ☐Shallow, ☐↑ Insp effort, ☐↑ Exp effort
  - *Sounds/Localization*:
    - ☐Norm BV, ☐Quiet BV, ☐Loud BV, ☐Crack, ☐Wheez, ☐Frict, ☐Muffled
    - ☐All fields, ☐Rt cran, ☐Rt mid, ☐Rt caud, ☐Lt cran, ☐Lt mid, ☐Lt caud
  - *Tracheal Auscultation/ Palpation*: ☐Normal, Other:_____

- **Pain Score**:_____ / 5   Localization:_____

- **Mentation**: ☐BAR   ☐Confused/   ☐Drowsy/   ☐Stuporous   ☐Coma
         ☐QAR   Disoriented   Obtunded   (unresponsive
         ☐Dull   unless aroused by
                                           noxious stimuli)

- **Skin Elasticity**: ☐Normal skin turgor, ☐↓ Skin turgor, ☐Skin tent, ☐Gelatinous

- **Mucus Membranes**:
  - *CRT*:_____ [*RI*: 1–2; <1 = compensated shock, sepsis, heat stroke; <2 = acute decompensated shock; >2 = late decompensated shock, decreased cardiac output, hypothermia]
  - *Color*:_____ [*RI*: pink; red = compensated shock, sepsis, heat stroke; pale/white = anemia, shock; blue = cyanosis; yellow = hepatic disease, extravascular hemolysis; brown = met-Hb]
  - *Texture*:_____ [*RI*: moist = hydrated; tacky-to-dry = 5–12% dehydrated]

Physical Exam – Systems Checklist:

- Head:_____ ☐NAF
  - Ears: ☐Debris (mild / mod / sev) (AS / AD / AU),_____ ☐NAF
  - Eyes:_____ ☐NAF
    - Retinal:_____ ☐NAF

	→ ⊙ L		⊙ R		⊙ L		⊙ R ←
☐	Normal Direct	☐	Normal Indirect	☐	Normal Indirect	☐	Normal Direct
☐	Abnormal Direct	☐	Abnormal Indirect	☐	Abnormal Indirect	☐	Abnormal Direct

  - Nose:_____ ☐NAF
  - Oral cavity: ☐Tarter/Gingivitis (mild / mod / sev),_____ ☐NAF
  - Mandibular lnn.: ☐Enlarged Lt., ☐Enlarged Rt.,_____ ☐NAF

- Neck:_____ ☐NAF
  - Superficial cervical lnn.: ☐Enlarged Lt., ☐Enlarged Rt.,_____ ☐NAF
  - Thyroid:_____ ☐NAF

- Thoracic limb:_____ ☐NAF
  - Foot pads:_____ ☐NAF
  - Knuckling:_____ ☐NAF
  - Axillary lnn. [normally absent]:_____ ☐NAF

- Thorax:_____ ☐NAF

- Abdomen:_____ ☐NAF
  - Mammary chain:_____ ☐NAF
  - Penis/ Testicles/ Vulva:_____ ☐NAF
  - Superficial inguinal lnn. [normally absent]:_____ ☐NAF

- Pelvic limb:_____ ☐NAF
  - Foot pads:_____ ☐NAF
  - Knuckling:_____ ☐NAF
  - Popliteal lnn.: ☐Enlarged Lt., ☐Enlarged Rt.,_____ ☐NAF

- Skin:_____ ☐NAF
- Tail:_____ ☐NAF
- Rectal☞ ☉:_____ ☐NAF

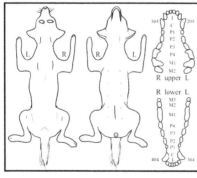

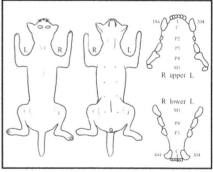

Problems List:

• **Problem #1**:

• **Problem #2**:

• **Problem #3**:

• **Problem #4**:

• **Problem #5**:

Diagnostic Plan	Treatment Plan

Case No._____

Patient	Age	Sex	Breed	Weight
	DOB:	Mn / Mi Fs / Fi	Color:	kg

Owner		Primary Veterinarian	Admit Date/ Time
Name: Phone:		Name: Phone:	Date: Time: AM / PM

• **Presenting Complaint**:_____
_____
_____

• **Medical Hx**:_____
_____
_____

• **When/ where obtained**: Date:_____; ☐Breeder, ☐Shelter, Other:_____

Drug/ Suppl.	Amount	Dose (mg/kg)	Route	Frequency	Date Started

• **Vaccine status – Dog**: ☐Rab ☐Parv ☐Dist ☐Aden; ☐Para ☐Lep ☐Bord ☐Influ ☐Lyme
• **Vaccine status – Cat**: ☐Rab ☐Herp ☐Cali ☐Pan ☐FeLV[kittens]; ☐FIV ☐Chlam ☐Bord
• **Heartworm / Flea & Tick / Intestinal Parasites**:
  ◦ *Last Heartworm Test*: Date:_____, ☐IDK; Test Results: ☐Pos, ☐Neg, ☐IDK
  ◦ *Monthly heartworm preventative*: ☐no ☐yes, Product:_____
  ◦ *Monthly flea & tick preventative*: ☐no ☐yes, Product:_____
  ◦ *Monthly dewormer*: ☐no ☐yes, Product:_____
• **Surgical Hx**: ☐Spay/Neuter; Date:_____; Other:_____
• **Environment**: ☐Indoor, ☐Outdoor, Time spent outdoors/ Other:_____
• **Housemates**: Dogs:_____ Cats:_____ Other:_____
• **Diet**: ☐Wet, ☐Dry; Brand/ Amt.:_____

Appetite	☐Normal, ☐↑, ☐↓
Weight	☐Normal, ☐↑, ☐↓; Past Wt.:_____ kg; Date:_____; Δ:_____
Thirst	☐Normal, ☐↑, ☐↓
Urination	☐Normal, ☐↑, ☐↓, ☐Blood, ☐Strain
Defecation	☐Normal, ☐↑, ☐↓, ☐Blood, ☐Strain, ☐Diarrhea, ☐Mucus
Discharge	☐No, ☐Yes; Onset/ Describe:
Cough/ Sneeze	☐No, ☐Yes; Onset/ Describe:
Vomit	☐No, ☐Yes; Onset/ Describe:
Respiration	☐Normal, ☐↑ Rate, ☐↑ Effort
Energy level	☐Normal, ☐Lethargic, ☐Exercise intolerance

• **Travel Hx**: ☐None, Other:_____
• **Exposure to**: ☐Standing water, ☐Wildlife, ☐Board/daycare, ☐Dog park, ☐Groomer
• **Adverse reactions to food/ meds**: ☐None, Other:_____
• **Can give oral meds**: ☐no ☐yes; Helpful Tricks:_____

Physical Exam – General:

• **Body Weight**:_____kg   **Body Condition Score**:_____/9

• **Temperature**:_____°F [*Dog-RI*: 100.9–102.4; *Cat-RI*: 98.1–102.1]

• **Heart**:
   ○ *Rate*:_____beats/min [Dog-RI: 60–180; Cat-RI: 140–240 (in hospital)]
   ○ *Rhythm*:   ☐Regular, ☐Irregular
   ○ *Sounds*:   ☐None, ☐Split sound, ☐Gallop, ☐Murmur, ☐Muffled
     ▪ *Grade*:   ☐1–2[soft, only at PMI],   ☐3–4[moderate, mild radiate],   ☐5–6[strong radiate, thrill]
     ▪ *Timing*: ☐Systolic, ☐Diastolic, ☐Continuous
     ▪ *PMI*:

	PMI	Over	Anatomic Boundaries
☐	Lt. apex	Mitral valve	5th to 6th ICS at level of CCJ
☐	Lt. base	Ao + Pul outflow	2nd to 4th ICS above the CCJ
☐	Rt. midheart	Tricuspid valve	3rd to 5th ICS near the CCJ
☐	Rt. sternal border	Right ventricle	5th to 7th ICS immediately dorsal to the sternum
☐	Sternal (cat)	Sternum	In cats, PMI offers very little clinical significance.

    •   *Vertebral Heart Size*: Dog = 8.7–10.5; Cat = 6.9–8.1 (from cranial edge of T4)
    •   *Innocent Murmur*: Grade 1-2, systolic, left base location, disappear by ~4 months of age, absent clinical signs

• **Pulses**:
   ○ *Pulse rate*:_____pulses/min
   ○ *Character*:   ☐Sync, ☐Async;   ☐Normokinetic, ☐Hyper-, ☐Hypo-, ☐Variable

• **Lungs**:
   ○ *Respiratory rate*:_____breaths/min [*RI*: 16–30]
   ○ *Depth/Effort*: ☐Norm, ☐Pant, ☐Deep, ☐Shallow, ☐↑ Insp effort, ☐↑ Exp effort
   ○ *Sounds/Localization*:
     ▪ ☐Norm BV, ☐Quiet BV, ☐Loud BV, ☐Crack, ☐Wheez, ☐Frict, ☐Muffled
     ▪ ☐All fields, ☐Rt cran, ☐Rt mid, ☐Rt caud, ☐Lt cran, ☐Lt mid, ☐Lt caud
   ○ *Tracheal Auscultation/ Palpation*: ☐Normal, Other:_____

• **Pain Score**:_____ / 5   Localization:_____

• **Mentation**: ☐BAR   ☐Confused/   ☐Drowsy/   ☐Stuporous   ☐Coma
                 ☐QAR   Disoriented   Obtunded   (unresponsive
                 ☐Dull   unless aroused by
                                                      noxious stimuli)

• **Skin Elasticity**: ☐Normal skin turgor, ☐↓ Skin turgor, ☐Skin tent, ☐Gelatinous

• **Mucus Membranes**:
   ○ *CRT*:_____ [*RI*: 1–2; <1 = compensated shock, sepsis, heat stroke; <2 = acute decompensated shock; >2 = late decompensated shock, decreased cardiac output, hypothermia]
   ○ *Color*:_____ [*RI*: pink; red = compensated shock, sepsis, heat stroke; pale/white = anemia, shock; blue = cyanosis; yellow = hepatic disease, extravascular hemolysis; brown = met-Hb]
   ○ *Texture*:_____ [*RI*: moist = hydrated; tacky-to-dry = 5–12% dehydrated]

<u>Physical Exam – Systems Checklist</u>:

- Head:_____ ☐NAF
  - Ears: ☐Debris (mild / mod / sev) (AS / AD / AU),_____ ☐NAF
  - Eyes:_____ ☐NAF
    - Retinal:_____ ☐NAF

	→ (L)		(R)		(L)		(R) ←
☐	Normal Direct	☐	Normal Indirect	☐	Normal Indirect	☐	Normal Direct
☐	Abnormal Direct	☐	Abnormal Indirect	☐	Abnormal Indirect	☐	Abnormal Direct

  - Nose:_____ ☐NAF
  - Oral cavity: ☐Tarter/Gingivitis (mild / mod / sev),_____ ☐NAF
  - Mandibular lnn.: ☐Enlarged Lt., ☐Enlarged Rt.,_____ ☐NAF

- Neck:_____ ☐NAF
  - Superficial cervical lnn.: ☐Enlarged Lt., ☐Enlarged Rt.,___ ☐NAF
  - Thyroid:_____ ☐NAF

- Thoracic limb:_____ ☐NAF
  - Foot pads:_____ ☐NAF
  - Knuckling:_____ ☐NAF
  - Axillary lnn. [normally absent]:_____ ☐NAF

- Thorax:_____ ☐NAF

- Abdomen:_____ ☐NAF
  - Mammary chain:_____ ☐NAF
  - Penis/ Testicles/ Vulva:_____ ☐NAF
  - Superficial inguinal lnn. [normally absent]:_____ ☐NAF

- Pelvic limb:_____ ☐NAF
  - Foot pads:_____ ☐NAF
  - Knuckling:_____ ☐NAF
  - Popliteal lnn.: ☐Enlarged Lt., ☐Enlarged Rt.,_____ ☐NAF

- Skin:_____ ☐NAF
- Tail:_____ ☐NAF
- Rectal☞⊙:_____ ☐NAF

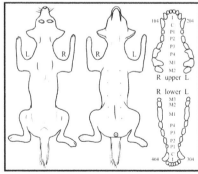
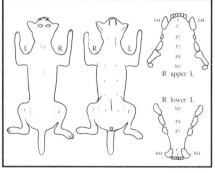

54

Problems List:

• **Problem #1**:

• **Problem #2**:

• **Problem #3**:

• **Problem #4**:

• **Problem #5**:

Diagnostic Plan	Treatment Plan

Case No._____

Patient	Age	Sex	Breed		Weight
	DOB:	Mn / Mi Fs / Fi	Color:		kg

Owner	Primary Veterinarian	Admit Date/ Time
Name: Phone:	Name: Phone:	Date: Time: AM / PM

• **Presenting Complaint**:_____
_____
_____

• **Medical Hx**:_____
_____
_____

• **When/ where obtained**:   Date:_____; □Breeder, □Shelter, Other:_____

Drug/ Suppl.	Amount	Dose (mg/kg)	Route	Frequency	Date Started

• **Vaccine status – Dog**: □Rab □Parv □Dist □Aden; □Para □Lep □Bord □Influ □Lyme
• **Vaccine status – Cat**: □Rab □Herp □Cali □Pan □FeLV[kittens]; □FIV □Chlam □Bord
• **Heartworm / Flea & Tick / Intestinal Parasites**:
   ◦ *Last Heartworm Test*: Date:_____, □IDK; Test Results: □Pos, □Neg, □IDK
   ◦ *Monthly heartworm preventative*: □no □yes, Product:_____
   ◦ *Monthly flea & tick preventative*: □no □yes, Product:_____
   ◦ *Monthly dewormer*: □no □yes, Product:_____
• **Surgical Hx**: □Spay/Neuter; Date:_____; Other:_____
• **Environment**: □Indoor, □Outdoor, Time spent outdoors/ Other:_____
• **Housemates**: Dogs:_____ Cats:_____ Other:_____
• **Diet**: □Wet, □Dry; Brand/ Amt.:_____

Appetite	□Normal, □↑, □↓
Weight	□Normal, □↑, □↓; Past Wt.:_____ kg; Date:_____; Δ:_____
Thirst	□Normal, □↑, □↓
Urination	□Normal, □↑, □↓, □Blood, □Strain
Defecation	□Normal, □↑, □↓, □Blood, □Strain, □Diarrhea, □Mucus
Discharge	□No, □Yes; Onset/ Describe:
Cough/ Sneeze	□No, □Yes; Onset/ Describe:
Vomit	□No, □Yes; Onset/ Describe:
Respiration	□Normal, □↑ Rate, □↑ Effort
Energy level	□Normal, □Lethargic, □Exercise intolerance

• **Travel Hx**: □None, Other:_____
• **Exposure to**: □Standing water, □Wildlife, □Board/daycare, □Dog park, □Groomer
• **Adverse reactions to food/ meds**: □None, Other:_____
• **Can give oral meds**: □no □yes; Helpful Tricks:_____

Physical Exam – General:

- **Body Weight**:_____kg   **Body Condition Score**:_____/9

- **Temperature**:_____°F [*Dog-RI*: 100.9–102.4; *Cat-RI*: 98.1–102.1]

- **Heart**:
  - *Rate*:_____beats/min [Dog-RI: 60–180; Cat-RI: 140–240 (in hospital)]
  - *Rhythm*: ☐Regular, ☐Irregular
  - *Sounds*: ☐None, ☐Split sound, ☐Gallop, ☐Murmur, ☐Muffled
    - *Grade*: ☐1–2[soft, only at PMI], ☐3–4[moderate, mild radiate], ☐5–6[strong radiate, thrill]
    - *Timing*: ☐Systolic, ☐Diastolic, ☐Continuous
    - *PMI*:

	PMI	Over	Anatomic Boundaries
☐	Lt. apex	Mitral valve	5th to 6th ICS at level of CCJ
☐	Lt. base	Ao + Pul outflow	2nd to 4th ICS above the CCJ
☐	Rt. midheart	Tricuspid valve	3rd to 5th ICS near the CCJ
☐	Rt. sternal border	Right ventricle	5th to 7th ICS immediately dorsal to the sternum
☐	Sternal (cat)	Sternum	In cats, PMI offers very little clinical significance.

  - *Vertebral Heart Size*: Dog = 8.7–10.5; Cat = 6.9–8.1 (from cranial edge of T4)
  - *Innocent Murmur*: Grade 1-2, systolic, left base location, disappear by ~4 months of age, absent clinical signs

- **Pulses**:
  - *Pulse rate*:_____pulses/min
  - *Character*: ☐Sync, ☐Async; ☐Normokinetic, ☐Hyper-, ☐Hypo-, ☐Variable

- **Lungs**:
  - *Respiratory rate*:_____breaths/min [*RI*: 16–30]
  - *Depth/Effort*: ☐Norm, ☐Pant, ☐Deep, ☐Shallow, ☐↑ Insp effort, ☐↑ Exp effort
  - *Sounds/Localization*:
    - ☐Norm BV, ☐Quiet BV, ☐Loud BV, ☐Crack, ☐Wheez, ☐Frict, ☐Muffled
    - ☐All fields, ☐Rt cran, ☐Rt mid, ☐Rt caud, ☐Lt cran, ☐Lt mid, ☐Lt caud
  - *Tracheal Auscultation/ Palpation*: ☐Normal, Other:_____

- **Pain Score**:_____ / 5   Localization:_____

- **Mentation**: ☐BAR   ☐Confused/   ☐Drowsy/   ☐Stuporous   ☐Coma
  ☐QAR   Disoriented   Obtunded   (unresponsive
  ☐Dull   unless aroused by
                                                        noxious stimuli)

- **Skin Elasticity**: ☐Normal skin turgor, ☐↓ Skin turgor, ☐Skin tent, ☐Gelatinous

- **Mucus Membranes**:
  - *CRT*:_____ [*RI*: 1–2; <1 = compensated shock, sepsis, heat stroke; <2 = acute decompensated shock; >2 = late decompensated shock, decreased cardiac output, hypothermia]
  - *Color*:_____ [*RI*: pink; red = compensated shock, sepsis, heat stroke; pale/white = anemia, shock; blue = cyanosis; yellow = hepatic disease, extravascular hemolysis; brown = met-Hb]
  - *Texture*:_____ [*RI*: moist = hydrated; tacky-to-dry = 5–12% dehydrated]

Physical Exam – Systems Checklist:

- Head:_____ ☐NAF
  - Ears: ☐Debris (mild / mod / sev) (AS / AD / AU),_____ ☐NAF
  - Eyes:_____ ☐NAF
    - Retinal:_____ ☐NAF

→ ⬤ L		⬤ R		⬤ L		⬤ R ←	
☐	Normal Direct	☐	Normal Indirect	☐	Normal Indirect	☐	Normal Direct
☐	Abnormal Direct	☐	Abnormal Indirect	☐	Abnormal Indirect	☐	Abnormal Direct

  - Nose:_____ ☐NAF
  - Oral cavity: ☐Tarter/Gingivitis (mild / mod / sev),_____ ☐NAF
  - Mandibular lnn.: ☐Enlarged Lt., ☐Enlarged Rt.,_____ ☐NAF

- Neck:_____ ☐NAF
  - Superficial cervical lnn.: ☐Enlarged Lt., ☐Enlarged Rt.,_____ ☐NAF
  - Thyroid:_____ ☐NAF

- Thoracic limb:_____ ☐NAF
  - Foot pads:_____ ☐NAF
  - Knuckling:_____ ☐NAF
  - Axillary lnn. [normally absent]:_____ ☐NAF

- Thorax:_____ ☐NAF

- Abdomen:_____ ☐NAF
  - Mammary chain:_____ ☐NAF
  - Penis/ Testicles/ Vulva:_____ ☐NAF
  - Superficial inguinal lnn. [normally absent]:_____ ☐NAF

- Pelvic limb:_____ ☐NAF
  - Foot pads:_____ ☐NAF
  - Knuckling:_____ ☐NAF
  - Popliteal lnn.: ☐Enlarged Lt., ☐Enlarged Rt.,_____ ☐NAF

- Skin:_____ ☐NAF
- Tail:_____ ☐NAF
- Rectal☞☉:_____ ☐NAF

<u>**Problems List**</u>:

• **Problem #1**:

• **Problem #2**:

• **Problem #3**:

• **Problem #4**:

• **Problem #5**:

Diagnostic Plan	Treatment Plan

Case No._____

Patient	Age	Sex	Breed	Weight
	DOB:	Mn / Mi Fs / Fi	Color:	kg

Owner	Primary Veterinarian	Admit Date/ Time
Name: Phone:	Name: Phone:	Date: Time: AM / PM

• **Presenting Complaint**:_____
_____
_____

• **Medical Hx**:_____
_____
_____

• **When/ where obtained**:   Date:_____ ; □Breeder, □Shelter, Other:_____

Drug/ Suppl.	Amount	Dose (mg/kg)	Route	Frequency	Date Started

• **Vaccine status – Dog**: □Rab □Parv □Dist □Aden; □Para □Lep □Bord □Influ □Lyme
• **Vaccine status – Cat**: □Rab □Herp □Cali □Pan □FeLV[kittens]; □FIV □Chlam □Bord
• **Heartworm / Flea & Tick / Intestinal Parasites**:
  ◦ *Last Heartworm Test*: Date:_____, □IDK; Test Results: □Pos, □Neg, □IDK
  ◦ *Monthly heartworm preventative*: □no □yes, Product:_____
  ◦ *Monthly flea & tick preventative*: □no □yes, Product:_____
  ◦ *Monthly dewormer*:   □no □yes, Product:_____
• **Surgical Hx**:   □Spay/Neuter; Date:_____ ; Other:_____
• **Environment**: □Indoor, □Outdoor, Time spent outdoors/ Other:_____
• **Housemates**: Dogs:_____ Cats:_____ Other:_____
• **Diet**: □Wet, □Dry; Brand/ Amt.:_____

Appetite	□Normal, □↑, □↓
Weight	□Normal, □↑, □↓; Past Wt.:_____ kg; Date:_____ ; Δ:_____
Thirst	□Normal, □↑, □↓
Urination	□Normal, □↑, □↓, □Blood, □Strain
Defecation	□Normal, □↑, □↓, □Blood, □Strain, □Diarrhea, □Mucus
Discharge	□No, □Yes; Onset/ Describe:
Cough/ Sneeze	□No, □Yes; Onset/ Describe:
Vomit	□No, □Yes; Onset/ Describe:
Respiration	□Normal, □↑ Rate, □↑ Effort
Energy level	□Normal, □Lethargic, □Exercise intolerance

• **Travel Hx**: □None, Other:_____
• **Exposure to**: □Standing water, □Wildlife, □Board/daycare, □Dog park, □Groomer
• **Adverse reactions to food/ meds**: □None, Other:_____
• **Can give oral meds**: □no □yes; Helpful Tricks:_____

Physical Exam – General:

- **Body Weight**:_____kg   **Body Condition Score**:_____/9

- **Temperature**:_____°F *[Dog-RI: 100.9–102.4; Cat-RI: 98.1–102.1]*

- **Heart**:
  - *Rate*:_____beats/min [Dog-RI: 60–180; Cat-RI: 140–240 (in hospital)]
  - *Rhythm*:   □Regular, □Irregular
  - *Sounds*:   □None, □Split sound, □Gallop, □Murmur, □Muffled
    - *Grade*:   □1–2[soft, only at PMI],   □3–4[moderate, mild radiate],   □5–6[strong radiate, thrill]
    - *Timing*: □Systolic, □Diastolic, □Continuous
    - *PMI*:

	PMI	Over	Anatomic Boundaries
□	Lt. apex	Mitral valve	5th to 6th ICS at level of CCJ
□	Lt. base	Ao + Pul outflow	2nd to 4th ICS above the CCJ
□	Rt. midheart	Tricuspid valve	3rd to 5th ICS near the CCJ
□	Rt. sternal border	Right ventricle	5th to 7th ICS immediately dorsal to the sternum
□	Sternal (cat)	Sternum	In cats, PMI offers very little clinical significance.

- *Vertebral Heart Size*: Dog = 8.7–10.5; Cat = 6.9–8.1 (from cranial edge of T4)
- *Innocent Murmur*: Grade 1-2, systolic, left base location, disappear by ~4 months of age, absent clinical signs

- **Pulses**:
  - *Pulse rate*:_____pulses/min
  - *Character*:   □Sync, □Async;   □Normokinetic, □Hyper-, □Hypo-, □Variable

- **Lungs**:
  - *Respiratory rate*:_____breaths/min [RI: 16–30]
  - *Depth/Effort*: □Norm, □Pant, □Deep, □Shallow, □↑ Insp effort, □↑ Exp effort
  - *Sounds/Localization*:
    - □Norm BV, □Quiet BV, □Loud BV, □Crack, □Wheez, □Frict, □Muffled
    - □All fields, □Rt cran, □Rt mid, □Rt caud, □Lt cran, □Lt mid, □Lt caud
  - *Tracheal Auscultation/ Palpation*: □Normal, Other:_____

- **Pain Score**:_____ / 5   Localization:_____

- **Mentation**: □BAR   □Confused/   □Drowsy/   □Stuporous   □Coma
                 □QAR   Disoriented   Obtunded   (unresponsive
                 □Dull   unless aroused by
                                                                     noxious stimuli)

- **Skin Elasticity**: □Normal skin turgor, □↓ Skin turgor, □Skin tent, □Gelatinous

- **Mucus Membranes**:
  - *CRT*:_____ [RI: 1–2; <1 = compensated shock, sepsis, heat stroke; <2 = acute decompensated shock; >2 = late decompensated shock, decreased cardiac output, hypothermia]
  - *Color*:_____ [RI: pink; red = compensated shock, sepsis, heat stroke; pale/white = anemia, shock; blue = cyanosis; yellow = hepatic disease, extravascular hemolysis; brown = met-Hb]
  - *Texture*:_____ [RI: moist = hydrated; tacky-to-dry = 5–12% dehydrated]

Physical Exam – Systems Checklist:

- Head:_____ ☐NAF
  - Ears: ☐Debris (mild / mod / sev) (AS / AD / AU),_____ ☐NAF
  - Eyes:_____ ☐NAF
    - Retinal:_____ ☐NAF

➔ Ⓛ	Ⓡ	Ⓛ	Ⓡ ⬅
☐ Normal Direct	☐ Normal Indirect	☐ Normal Indirect	☐ Normal Direct
☐ Abnormal Direct	☐ Abnormal Indirect	☐ Abnormal Indirect	☐ Abnormal Direct

  - Nose:_____ ☐NAF
  - Oral cavity: ☐Tarter/Gingivitis (mild / mod / sev),_____ ☐NAF
  - Mandibular lnn.: ☐Enlarged Lt., ☐Enlarged Rt.,_____ ☐NAF

- Neck:_____ ☐NAF
  - Superficial cervical lnn.: ☐Enlarged Lt., ☐Enlarged Rt.,_____ ☐NAF
  - Thyroid:_____ ☐NAF

- Thoracic limb:_____ ☐NAF
  - Foot pads:_____ ☐NAF
  - Knuckling:_____ ☐NAF
  - Axillary lnn. [normally absent]:_____ ☐NAF

- Thorax:_____ ☐NAF

- Abdomen:_____ ☐NAF
  - Mammary chain:_____ ☐NAF
  - Penis/ Testicles/ Vulva:_____ ☐NAF
  - Superficial inguinal lnn. [normally absent]:_____ ☐NAF

- Pelvic limb:_____ ☐NAF
  - Foot pads:_____ ☐NAF
  - Knuckling:_____ ☐NAF
  - Popliteal lnn.: ☐Enlarged Lt., ☐Enlarged Rt.,_____ ☐NAF

- Skin:_____ ☐NAF
- Tail:_____ ☐NAF
- Rectal☞☉:_____ ☐NAF

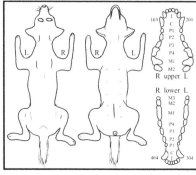
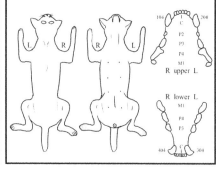

<u>**Problems List**</u>:

• **Problem #1**:

• **Problem #2**:

• **Problem #3**:

• **Problem #4**:

• **Problem #5**:

Diagnostic Plan	Treatment Plan

Case No._____

Patient		Age	Sex	Breed	Weight
		DOB:	Mn / Mi Fs / Fi	Color:	kg

Owner	Primary Veterinarian	Admit Date/ Time
Name: Phone:	Name: Phone:	Date: Time: AM / PM

• **Presenting Complaint**:_____
_____
_____

• **Medical Hx**:_____
_____
_____

• **When/ where obtained**: Date:_____; ☐Breeder, ☐Shelter, Other:_____

Drug/ Suppl.	Amount	Dose (mg/kg)	Route	Frequency	Date Started

• **Vaccine status – Dog**: ☐Rab ☐Parv ☐Dist ☐Aden; ☐Para ☐Lep ☐Bord ☐Influ ☐Lyme
• **Vaccine status – Cat**: ☐Rab ☐Herp ☐Cali ☐Pan ☐FeLV[kittens]; ☐FIV ☐Chlam ☐Bord
• **Heartworm / Flea & Tick / Intestinal Parasites**:
    ◦ *Last Heartworm Test*: Date:_____, ☐IDK; Test Results: ☐Pos, ☐Neg, ☐IDK
    ◦ *Monthly heartworm preventative*:   ☐no ☐yes, Product:_____
    ◦ *Monthly flea & tick preventative*:   ☐no ☐yes, Product:_____
    ◦ *Monthly dewormer*:   ☐no ☐yes, Product:_____
• **Surgical Hx**:   ☐Spay/Neuter; Date:_____; Other:_____
• **Environment**: ☐Indoor, ☐Outdoor, Time spent outdoors/ Other:_____
• **Housemates**: Dogs:_____ Cats:_____ Other:_____
• **Diet**: ☐Wet, ☐Dry; Brand/ Amt.:_____

Appetite	☐Normal, ☐↑, ☐↓
Weight	☐Normal, ☐↑, ☐↓; Past Wt.:_____ kg; Date:_____; Δ:_____
Thirst	☐Normal, ☐↑, ☐↓
Urination	☐Normal, ☐↑, ☐↓, ☐Blood, ☐Strain
Defecation	☐Normal, ☐↑, ☐↓, ☐Blood, ☐Strain, ☐Diarrhea, ☐Mucus
Discharge	☐No, ☐Yes; Onset/ Describe:
Cough/ Sneeze	☐No, ☐Yes; Onset/ Describe:
Vomit	☐No, ☐Yes; Onset/ Describe:
Respiration	☐Normal, ☐↑ Rate, ☐↑ Effort
Energy level	☐Normal, ☐Lethargic, ☐Exercise intolerance

• **Travel Hx**: ☐None, Other:_____
• **Exposure to**: ☐Standing water, ☐Wildlife, ☐Board/daycare, ☐Dog park, ☐Groomer
• **Adverse reactions to food/ meds**: ☐None, Other:_____
• **Can give oral meds**: ☐no ☐yes; Helpful Tricks:_____

Physical Exam – General:

- **Body Weight**:_____kg **Body Condition Score**:_____/9

- **Temperature**:_____°F [*Dog-RI*: 100.9–102.4; *Cat-RI*: 98.1–102.1]

- **Heart**:
  - *Rate*:_____beats/min [Dog-RI: 60–180; Cat-RI: 140–240 (in hospital)]
  - *Rhythm*: □Regular, □Irregular
  - *Sounds*: □None, □Split sound, □Gallop, □Murmur, □Muffled
    - *Grade*: □1–2[soft, only at PMI], □3–4[moderate, mild radiate], □5–6[strong radiate, thrill]
    - *Timing*: □Systolic, □Diastolic, □Continuous
    - *PMI*:

	PMI	Over	Anatomic Boundaries
□	Lt. apex	Mitral valve	5th to 6th ICS at level of CCJ
□	Lt. base	Ao + Pul outflow	2nd to 4th ICS above the CCJ
□	Rt. midheart	Tricuspid valve	3rd to 5th ICS near the CCJ
□	Rt. sternal border	Right ventricle	5th to 7th ICS immediately dorsal to the sternum
□	Sternal (cat)	Sternum	In cats, PMI offers very little clinical significance.

  - *Vertebral Heart Size*: Dog = 8.7–10.5; Cat = 6.9–8.1 (from cranial edge of T4)
  - *Innocent Murmur*: Grade 1-2, systolic, left base location, disappear by ~4 months of age, absent clinical signs

- **Pulses**:
  - *Pulse rate*:_____pulses/min
  - *Character*: □Sync, □Async; □Normokinetic, □Hyper-, □Hypo-, □Variable

- **Lungs**:
  - *Respiratory rate*:_____breaths/min [*RI*: 16–30]
  - *Depth/Effort*: □Norm, □Pant, □Deep, □Shallow, □↑ Insp effort, □↑ Exp effort
  - *Sounds/Localization*:
    - □Norm BV, □Quiet BV, □Loud BV, □Crack, □Wheez, □Frict, □Muffled
    - □All fields, □Rt cran, □Rt mid, □Rt caud, □Lt cran, □Lt mid, □Lt caud
  - *Tracheal Auscultation/ Palpation*: □Normal, Other:_____

- **Pain Score**:_____ / 5   Localization:_____

- **Mentation**: □BAR   □Confused/   □Drowsy/   □Stuporous   □Coma
  □QAR   Disoriented   Obtunded   (unresponsive
  □Dull   unless aroused by
  noxious stimuli)

- **Skin Elasticity**: □Normal skin turgor, □↓ Skin turgor, □Skin tent, □Gelatinous

- **Mucus Membranes**:
  - *CRT*:_____ [*RI*: 1–2; <1 = compensated shock, sepsis, heat stroke; <2 = acute decompensated shock; >2 = late decompensated shock, decreased cardiac output, hypothermia]
  - *Color*:_____ [*RI*: pink; red = compensated shock, sepsis, heat stroke; pale/white = anemia, shock; blue = cyanosis; yellow = hepatic disease, extravascular hemolysis; brown = met-Hb]
  - *Texture*:_____ [*RI*: moist = hydrated; tacky-to-dry = 5–12% dehydrated]

Physical Exam – Systems Checklist:

- Head:_____ ☐NAF
  - Ears: ☐Debris (mild / mod / sev) (AS / AD / AU), _____ ☐NAF
  - Eyes:_____ ☐NAF
    - Retinal:_____ ☐NAF

→ Ⓛ	Ⓡ	Ⓛ	Ⓡ ←
☐ Normal Direct	☐ Normal Indirect	☐ Normal Indirect	☐ Normal Direct
☐ Abnormal Direct	☐ Abnormal Indirect	☐ Abnormal Indirect	☐ Abnormal Direct

  - Nose:_____ ☐NAF
  - Oral cavity: ☐Tarter/Gingivitis (mild / mod / sev), _____ ☐NAF
  - Mandibular lnn.: ☐Enlarged Lt., ☐Enlarged Rt., _____ ☐NAF

- Neck:_____ ☐NAF
  - Superficial cervical lnn.: ☐Enlarged Lt., ☐Enlarged Rt., _____ ☐NAF
  - Thyroid:_____ ☐NAF

- Thoracic limb:_____ ☐NAF
  - Foot pads:_____ ☐NAF
  - Knuckling:_____ ☐NAF
  - Axillary lnn. [normally absent]:_____ ☐NAF

- Thorax:_____ ☐NAF

- Abdomen:_____ ☐NAF
  - Mammary chain:_____ ☐NAF
  - Penis/ Testicles/ Vulva:_____ ☐NAF
  - Superficial inguinal lnn. [normally absent]:_____ ☐NAF

- Pelvic limb:_____ ☐NAF
  - Foot pads:_____ ☐NAF
  - Knuckling:_____ ☐NAF
  - Popliteal lnn.: ☐Enlarged Lt., ☐Enlarged Rt., _____ ☐NAF

- Skin:_____ ☐NAF
- Tail:_____ ☐NAF
- Rectal☞☉:_____ ☐NAF

Problems List:

- **Problem #1**:

- **Problem #2**:

- **Problem #3**:

- **Problem #4**:

- **Problem #5**:

Diagnostic Plan	Treatment Plan

Case No._____

Patient	Age	Sex	Breed	Weight
	DOB:	Mn / Mi Fs / Fi	Color:	kg

Owner	Primary Veterinarian	Admit Date/ Time
Name: Phone:	Name: Phone:	Date: Time: AM / PM

• **Presenting Complaint**:_____
_____
_____

• **Medical Hx**:_____
_____
_____

• **When/ where obtained**:   Date:_____; □Breeder, □Shelter, Other:_____

Drug/ Suppl.	Amount	Dose (mg/kg)	Route	Frequency	Date Started

• **Vaccine status – Dog**: □Rab □Parv □Dist □Aden; □Para □Lep □Bord □Influ □Lyme
• **Vaccine status – Cat**: □Rab □Herp □Cali □Pan □FeLV[kittens]; □FIV □Chlam □Bord
• **Heartworm / Flea & Tick / Intestinal Parasites**:
  ◦ *Last Heartworm Test*: Date:_____, □IDK; Test Results: □Pos, □Neg, □IDK
  ◦ *Monthly heartworm preventative*: □no □yes, Product:_____
  ◦ *Monthly flea & tick preventative*: □no □yes, Product:_____
  ◦ *Monthly dewormer*: □no □yes, Product:_____
• **Surgical Hx**: □Spay/Neuter; Date:_____; Other:_____
• **Environment**: □Indoor, □Outdoor, Time spent outdoors/ Other:_____
• **Housemates**: Dogs:_____ Cats:_____ Other:_____
• **Diet**: □Wet, □Dry; Brand/ Amt.:_____

Appetite	□Normal, □↑, □↓
Weight	□Normal, □↑, □↓; Past Wt.:_____ kg; Date:_____; Δ:_____
Thirst	□Normal, □↑, □↓
Urination	□Normal, □↑, □↓, □Blood, □Strain
Defecation	□Normal, □↑, □↓, □Blood, □Strain, □Diarrhea, □Mucus
Discharge	□No, □Yes; Onset/ Describe:
Cough/ Sneeze	□No, □Yes; Onset/ Describe:
Vomit	□No, □Yes; Onset/ Describe:
Respiration	□Normal, □↑ Rate, □↑ Effort
Energy level	□Normal, □Lethargic, □Exercise intolerance

• **Travel Hx**: □None, Other:_____
• **Exposure to**: □Standing water, □Wildlife, □Board/daycare, □Dog park, □Groomer
• **Adverse reactions to food/ meds**: □None, Other:_____
• **Can give oral meds**: □no □yes; Helpful Tricks:_____

Physical Exam – General:

- **Body Weight**:_____kg   **Body Condition Score**:_____/9

- **Temperature**:_____°F [*Dog-RI*: 100.9–102.4; *Cat-RI*: 98.1–102.1]

- **Heart**:
    - ◦ *Rate*:_____beats/min [Dog-RI: 60–180; Cat-RI: 140–240 (in hospital)]
    - ◦ *Rhythm*:   □Regular, □Irregular
    - ◦ *Sounds*:   □None, □Split sound, □Gallop, □Murmur, □Muffled
        - ▪ *Grade*:   □1–2[soft, only at PMI],   □3–4[moderate, mild radiate],   □5–6[strong radiate, thrill]
        - ▪ *Timing*: □Systolic, □Diastolic, □Continuous
        - ▪ *PMI*:

	PMI	Over	Anatomic Boundaries
□	Lt. apex	Mitral valve	5th to 6th ICS at level of CCJ
□	Lt. base	Ao + Pul outflow	2nd to 4th ICS above the CCJ
□	Rt. midheart	Tricuspid valve	3rd to 5th ICS near the CCJ
□	Rt. sternal border	Right ventricle	5th to 7th ICS immediately dorsal to the sternum
□	Sternal (cat)	Sternum	In cats, PMI offers very little clinical significance.

    - • *Vertebral Heart Size*: Dog = 8.7–10.5; Cat = 6.9–8.1 (from cranial edge of T4)
    - • *Innocent Murmur*: Grade 1-2, systolic, left base location, disappear by ~4 months of age, absent clinical signs

- **Pulses**:
    - ◦ *Pulse rate*:_____pulses/min
    - ◦ *Character*:   □Sync, □Async;   □Normokinetic, □Hyper-, □Hypo-, □Variable

- **Lungs**:
    - ◦ *Respiratory rate*:_____breaths/min [*RI*: 16–30]
    - ◦ *Depth/Effort*: □Norm, □Pant, □Deep, □Shallow, □↑ Insp effort, □↑ Exp effort
    - ◦ *Sounds/Localization*:
        - ▪ □Norm BV, □Quiet BV, □Loud BV, □Crack, □Wheez, □Frict, □Muffled
        - ▪ □All fields, □Rt cran, □Rt mid, □Rt caud, □Lt cran, □Lt mid, □Lt caud
    - ◦ *Tracheal Auscultation/ Palpation*: □Normal, Other:_____

- **Pain Score**:_____ / 5   Localization:_____

- **Mentation**: □BAR   □Confused/   □Drowsy/   □Stuporous   □Coma
                 □QAR   Disoriented   Obtunded   (unresponsive
                 □Dull   unless aroused by
                                                               noxious stimuli)

- **Skin Elasticity**: □Normal skin turgor, □↓ Skin turgor, □Skin tent, □Gelatinous

- **Mucus Membranes**:
    - ◦ *CRT*:_____ [*RI*: 1–2; <1 = compensated shock, sepsis, heat stroke; <2 = acute decompensated shock; >2 = late decompensated shock, decreased cardiac output, hypothermia]
    - ◦ *Color*:_____ [*RI*: pink; red = compensated shock, sepsis, heat stroke; pale/white = anemia, shock; blue = cyanosis; yellow = hepatic disease, extravascular hemolysis; brown = met-Hb]
    - ◦ *Texture*:_____ [*RI*: moist = hydrated; tacky-to-dry = 5–12% dehydrated]

Physical Exam – Systems Checklist:

- Head:_____ ☐NAF
  - Ears: ☐Debris (mild / mod / sev) (AS / AD / AU), _____ ☐NAF
  - Eyes:_____ ☐NAF
    - Retinal:_____ ☐NAF

→●L		●R		●L		●R ←	
☐	Normal Direct	☐	Normal Indirect	☐	Normal Indirect	☐	Normal Direct
☐	Abnormal Direct	☐	Abnormal Indirect	☐	Abnormal Indirect	☐	Abnormal Direct

  - Nose:_____ ☐NAF
  - Oral cavity: ☐Tarter/Gingivitis (mild / mod / sev), _____ ☐NAF
  - Mandibular lnn.: ☐Enlarged Lt., ☐Enlarged Rt., _____ ☐NAF

- Neck:_____ ☐NAF
  - Superficial cervical lnn.: ☐Enlarged Lt., ☐Enlarged Rt., _____ ☐NAF
  - Thyroid:_____ ☐NAF

- Thoracic limb:_____ ☐NAF
  - Foot pads:_____ ☐NAF
  - Knuckling:_____ ☐NAF
  - Axillary lnn. [normally absent]:_____ ☐NAF

- Thorax:_____ ☐NAF

- Abdomen:_____ ☐NAF
  - Mammary chain:_____ ☐NAF
  - Penis/ Testicles/ Vulva:_____ ☐NAF
  - Superficial inguinal lnn. [normally absent]:_____ ☐NAF

- Pelvic limb:_____ ☐NAF
  - Foot pads:_____ ☐NAF
  - Knuckling:_____ ☐NAF
  - Popliteal lnn.: ☐Enlarged Lt., ☐Enlarged Rt., _____ ☐NAF

- Skin:_____ ☐NAF
- Tail:_____ ☐NAF
- Rectal☞☉:_____ ☐NAF

Problems List:

• **Problem #1**:

• **Problem #2**:

• **Problem #3**:

• **Problem #4**:

• **Problem #5**:

Diagnostic Plan	Treatment Plan

Case No._____

Patient	Age	Sex	Breed	Weight
	DOB:	Mn / Mi Fs / Fi	Color:	kg

Owner	Primary Veterinarian	Admit Date/ Time
Name: Phone:	Name: Phone:	Date: Time: AM / PM

• **Presenting Complaint**:_____

_____

• **Medical Hx**:_____

_____

• **When/ where obtained**: Date:_____; ☐Breeder, ☐Shelter, Other:_____

Drug/ Suppl.	Amount	Dose (mg/kg)	Route	Frequency	Date Started

• **Vaccine status – Dog**: ☐Rab ☐Parv ☐Dist ☐Aden; ☐Para ☐Lep ☐Bord ☐Influ ☐Lyme
• **Vaccine status – Cat**: ☐Rab ☐Herp ☐Cali ☐Pan ☐FeLV[kittens]; ☐FIV ☐Chlam ☐Bord
• **Heartworm / Flea & Tick / Intestinal Parasites**:
   ◦ *Last Heartworm Test*: Date:_____, ☐IDK; Test Results: ☐Pos, ☐Neg, ☐IDK
   ◦ *Monthly heartworm preventative*: ☐no ☐yes, Product:_____
   ◦ *Monthly flea & tick preventative*: ☐no ☐yes, Product:_____
   ◦ *Monthly dewormer*: ☐no ☐yes, Product:_____
• **Surgical Hx**: ☐Spay/Neuter; Date:_____; Other:_____
• **Environment**: ☐Indoor, ☐Outdoor, Time spent outdoors/ Other:_____
• **Housemates**: Dogs:_____ Cats:_____ Other:_____
• **Diet**: ☐Wet, ☐Dry; Brand/ Amt.:_____

Appetite	☐Normal, ☐↑, ☐↓
Weight	☐Normal, ☐↑, ☐↓; Past Wt.:_____ kg; Date:_____; Δ:_____
Thirst	☐Normal, ☐↑, ☐↓
Urination	☐Normal, ☐↑, ☐↓, ☐Blood, ☐Strain
Defecation	☐Normal, ☐↑, ☐↓, ☐Blood, ☐Strain, ☐Diarrhea, ☐Mucus
Discharge	☐No, ☐Yes; Onset/ Describe:
Cough/ Sneeze	☐No, ☐Yes; Onset/ Describe:
Vomit	☐No, ☐Yes; Onset/ Describe:
Respiration	☐Normal, ☐↑ Rate, ☐↑ Effort
Energy level	☐Normal, ☐Lethargic, ☐Exercise intolerance

• **Travel Hx**: ☐None, Other:_____
• **Exposure to**: ☐Standing water, ☐Wildlife, ☐Board/daycare, ☐Dog park, ☐Groomer
• **Adverse reactions to food/ meds**: ☐None, Other:_____
• **Can give oral meds**: ☐no ☐yes; Helpful Tricks:_____

Physical Exam – General:

- **Body Weight**:_____kg   **Body Condition Score**:_____/9

- **Temperature**:_____°F [*Dog-RI*: 100.9–102.4; *Cat-RI*: 98.1–102.1]

- **Heart**:
  - *Rate*:_____beats/min [Dog-RI: 60–180; Cat-RI: 140–240 (in hospital)]
  - *Rhythm*: ☐Regular, ☐Irregular
  - *Sounds*: ☐None, ☐Split sound, ☐Gallop, ☐Murmur, ☐Muffled
    - *Grade*: ☐1–2[soft, only at PMI], ☐3–4[moderate, mild radiate], ☐5–6[strong radiate, thrill]
    - *Timing*: ☐Systolic, ☐Diastolic, ☐Continuous
    - *PMI*:

	PMI	Over	Anatomic Boundaries
☐	Lt. apex	Mitral valve	5th to 6th ICS at level of CCJ
☐	Lt. base	Ao + Pul outflow	2nd to 4th ICS above the CCJ
☐	Rt. midheart	Tricuspid valve	3rd to 5th ICS near the CCJ
☐	Rt. sternal border	Right ventricle	5th to 7th ICS immediately dorsal to the sternum
☐	Sternal (cat)	Sternum	In cats, PMI offers very little clinical significance.

- •   *Vertebral Heart Size*: Dog = 8.7–10.5; Cat = 6.9–8.1 (from cranial edge of T4)
- •   *Innocent Murmur*: Grade 1-2, systolic, left base location, disappear by ~4 months of age, absent clinical signs

- **Pulses**:
  - *Pulse rate*:_____pulses/min
  - *Character*: ☐Sync, ☐Async; ☐Normokinetic, ☐Hyper-, ☐Hypo-, ☐Variable

- **Lungs**:
  - *Respiratory rate*:_____breaths/min [*RI*: 16–30]
  - *Depth/Effort*: ☐Norm, ☐Pant, ☐Deep, ☐Shallow, ☐↑ Insp effort, ☐↑ Exp effort
  - *Sounds/Localization*:
    - ☐Norm BV, ☐Quiet BV, ☐Loud BV, ☐Crack, ☐Wheez, ☐Frict, ☐Muffled
    - ☐All fields, ☐Rt cran, ☐Rt mid, ☐Rt caud, ☐Lt cran, ☐Lt mid, ☐Lt caud
  - *Tracheal Auscultation/ Palpation*: ☐Normal, Other:_____

- **Pain Score**:_____ / 5   Localization:_____

- **Mentation**: ☐BAR   ☐Confused/   ☐Drowsy/   ☐Stuporous   ☐Coma
      ☐QAR   Disoriented   Obtunded   (unresponsive
      ☐Dull   unless aroused by
                                     noxious stimuli)

- **Skin Elasticity**: ☐Normal skin turgor, ☐↓ Skin turgor, ☐Skin tent, ☐Gelatinous

- **Mucus Membranes**:
  - *CRT*:_____ [*RI*: 1–2; <1 = compensated shock, sepsis, heat stroke; <2 = acute decompensated shock; >2 = late decompensated shock, decreased cardiac output, hypothermia]
  - *Color*:_____ [*RI*: pink; red = compensated shock, sepsis, heat stroke; pale/white = anemia, shock; blue = cyanosis; yellow = hepatic disease, extravascular hemolysis; brown = met-Hb]
  - *Texture*:_____ [*RI*: moist = hydrated; tacky-to-dry = 5–12% dehydrated]

Physical Exam – Systems Checklist:

- Head:_____ ☐NAF
  - Ears: ☐Debris (mild / mod / sev) (AS / AD / AU),_____ ☐NAF
  - Eyes:_____ ☐NAF
    - Retinal:_____ ☐NAF

	→ ◉		◉		◉		◉ ←
☐	Normal Direct	☐	Normal Indirect	☐	Normal Indirect	☐	Normal Direct
☐	Abnormal Direct	☐	Abnormal Indirect	☐	Abnormal Indirect	☐	Abnormal Direct

  - Nose:_____ ☐NAF
  - Oral cavity: ☐Tarter/Gingivitis (mild / mod / sev),_____ ☐NAF
  - Mandibular lnn.: ☐Enlarged Lt., ☐Enlarged Rt.,_____ ☐NAF

- Neck:_____ ☐NAF
  - Superficial cervical lnn.: ☐Enlarged Lt., ☐Enlarged Rt.,_____ ☐NAF
  - Thyroid:_____ ☐NAF

- Thoracic limb:_____ ☐NAF
  - Foot pads:_____ ☐NAF
  - Knuckling:_____ ☐NAF
  - Axillary lnn. [normally absent]:_____ ☐NAF

- Thorax:_____ ☐NAF

- Abdomen:_____ ☐NAF
  - Mammary chain:_____ ☐NAF
  - Penis/ Testicles/ Vulva:_____ ☐NAF
  - Superficial inguinal lnn. [normally absent]:_____ ☐NAF

- Pelvic limb:_____ ☐NAF
  - Foot pads:_____ ☐NAF
  - Knuckling:_____ ☐NAF
  - Popliteal lnn.: ☐Enlarged Lt., ☐Enlarged Rt.,_____ ☐NAF

- Skin:_____ ☐NAF
- Tail:_____ ☐NAF
- Rectal☞☉:_____ ☐NAF

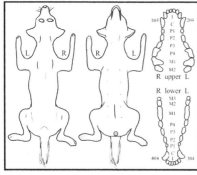
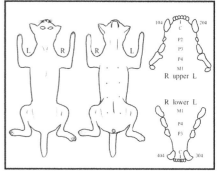

Problems List:

• **Problem #1**:

• **Problem #2**:

• **Problem #3**:

• **Problem #4**:

• **Problem #5**:

Diagnostic Plan	Treatment Plan

Case No._____

Patient	Age	Sex	Breed	Weight
	DOB:	Mn / Mi Fs / Fi	Color:	kg

Owner	Primary Veterinarian	Admit Date/ Time
Name: Phone:	Name: Phone:	Date: Time: AM / PM

• **Presenting Complaint**:_____

_____

• **Medical Hx**:_____

_____

• **When/ where obtained**:   Date:_____; ☐Breeder, ☐Shelter, Other:_____

Drug/ Suppl.	Amount	Dose (mg/kg)	Route	Frequency	Date Started

• **Vaccine status – Dog**: ☐Rab ☐Parv ☐Dist ☐Aden; ☐Para ☐Lep ☐Bord ☐Influ ☐Lyme
• **Vaccine status – Cat**: ☐Rab ☐Herp ☐Cali ☐Pan ☐FeLV[kittens]; ☐FIV ☐Chlam ☐Bord
• **Heartworm / Flea & Tick / Intestinal Parasites**:
   ◦ *Last Heartworm Test*: Date:_____, ☐IDK; Test Results: ☐Pos, ☐Neg, ☐IDK
   ◦ *Monthly heartworm preventative*: ☐no ☐yes, Product:_____
   ◦ *Monthly flea & tick preventative*: ☐no ☐yes, Product:_____
   ◦ *Monthly dewormer*:   ☐no ☐yes, Product:_____
• **Surgical Hx**:   ☐Spay/Neuter; Date:_____; Other:_____
• **Environment**: ☐Indoor, ☐Outdoor, Time spent outdoors/ Other:_____
• **Housemates**: Dogs:_____ Cats:_____ Other:_____
• **Diet**: ☐Wet, ☐Dry; Brand/ Amt.:_____

Appetite	☐Normal, ☐↑, ☐↓
Weight	☐Normal, ☐↑, ☐↓; Past Wt.:_____ kg; Date:_____; Δ:_____
Thirst	☐Normal, ☐↑, ☐↓
Urination	☐Normal, ☐↑, ☐↓, ☐Blood, ☐Strain
Defecation	☐Normal, ☐↑, ☐↓, ☐Blood, ☐Strain, ☐Diarrhea, ☐Mucus
Discharge	☐No, ☐Yes; Onset/ Describe:
Cough/ Sneeze	☐No, ☐Yes; Onset/ Describe:
Vomit	☐No, ☐Yes; Onset/ Describe:
Respiration	☐Normal, ☐↑ Rate, ☐↑ Effort
Energy level	☐Normal, ☐Lethargic, ☐Exercise intolerance

• **Travel Hx**: ☐None, Other:_____
• **Exposure to**: ☐Standing water, ☐Wildlife, ☐Board/daycare, ☐Dog park, ☐Groomer
• **Adverse reactions to food/ meds**: ☐None, Other:_____
• **Can give oral meds**: ☐no ☐yes; Helpful Tricks:_____

Physical Exam – General:

• **Body Weight**:_____kg   **Body Condition Score**:_____/9

• **Temperature**:_____°F [*Dog-RI*: 100.9–102.4; *Cat-RI*: 98.1–102.1]

• **Heart**:
  ○ *Rate*:_____beats/min [Dog-RI: 60–180; Cat-RI: 140–240 (in hospital)]
  ○ *Rhythm*:   □Regular, □Irregular
  ○ *Sounds*:   □None, □Split sound, □Gallop, □Murmur, □Muffled
    ▪ *Grade*:   □1–2[soft, only at PMI],   □3–4[moderate, mild radiate],   □5–6[strong radiate, thrill]
    ▪ *Timing*: □Systolic, □Diastolic, □Continuous
    ▪ *PMI*:

	PMI	Over	Anatomic Boundaries
□	Lt. apex	Mitral valve	5th to 6th ICS at level of CCJ
□	Lt. base	Ao + Pul outflow	2nd to 4th ICS above the CCJ
□	Rt. midheart	Tricuspid valve	3rd to 5th ICS near the CCJ
□	Rt. sternal border	Right ventricle	5th to 7th ICS immediately dorsal to the sternum
□	Sternal (cat)	Sternum	In cats, PMI offers very little clinical significance.

  - • *Vertebral Heart Size*: Dog = 8.7–10.5; Cat = 6.9–8.1 (from cranial edge of T4)
  - • *Innocent Murmur*: Grade 1-2, systolic, left base location, disappear by ~4 months of age, absent clinical signs

• **Pulses**:
  ○ *Pulse rate*:_____pulses/min
  ○ *Character*:   □Sync, □Async;   □Normokinetic, □Hyper-, □Hypo-, □Variable

• **Lungs**:
  ○ *Respiratory rate*:_____breaths/min [*RI*: 16–30]
  ○ *Depth/Effort*: □Norm, □Pant, □Deep, □Shallow, □↑ Insp effort, □↑ Exp effort
  ○ *Sounds/Localization*:
    ▪ □Norm BV, □Quiet BV, □Loud BV, □Crack, □Wheez, □Frict, □Muffled
    ▪ □All fields, □Rt cran, □Rt mid, □Rt caud, □Lt cran, □Lt mid, □Lt caud
  ○ *Tracheal Auscultation/ Palpation*: □Normal, Other:_____

• **Pain Score**:_____ / 5   Localization:_____

• **Mentation**: □BAR   □Confused/   □Drowsy/   □Stuporous   □Coma
                  □QAR   Disoriented   Obtunded   (unresponsive
                  □Dull   unless aroused by
                                                          noxious stimuli)

• **Skin Elasticity**: □Normal skin turgor, □↓ Skin turgor, □Skin tent, □Gelatinous

• **Mucus Membranes**:
  ○ *CRT*:_____ [*RI*: 1–2; <1 = compensated shock, sepsis, heat stroke; <2 = acute decompensated shock; >2 = late decompensated shock, decreased cardiac output, hypothermia]
  ○ *Color*:_____ [*RI*: pink; red = compensated shock, sepsis, heat stroke; pale/white = anemia, shock; blue = cyanosis; yellow = hepatic disease, extravascular hemolysis; brown = met-Hb]
  ○ *Texture*:_____ [*RI*: moist = hydrated; tacky-to-dry = 5–12% dehydrated]

Physical Exam – Systems Checklist:

- Head:_____ ☐NAF
  - Ears: ☐Debris (mild / mod / sev) (AS / AD / AU),_____ ☐NAF
  - Eyes:_____ ☐NAF
    - Retinal:_____ ☐NAF

	→ ⓛ		ⓡ		ⓛ		ⓡ ←
☐	Normal Direct	☐	Normal Indirect	☐	Normal Indirect	☐	Normal Direct
☐	Abnormal Direct	☐	Abnormal Indirect	☐	Abnormal Indirect	☐	Abnormal Direct

  - Nose:_____ ☐NAF
  - Oral cavity: ☐Tarter/Gingivitis (mild / mod / sev),_____ ☐NAF
  - Mandibular lnn.: ☐Enlarged Lt., ☐Enlarged Rt.,_____ ☐NAF

- Neck:_____ ☐NAF
  - Superficial cervical lnn.: ☐Enlarged Lt., ☐Enlarged Rt.,_____ ☐NAF
  - Thyroid:_____ ☐NAF

- Thoracic limb:_____ ☐NAF
  - Foot pads:_____ ☐NAF
  - Knuckling:_____ ☐NAF
  - Axillary lnn. [normally absent]:_____ ☐NAF

- Thorax:_____ ☐NAF

- Abdomen:_____ ☐NAF
  - Mammary chain:_____ ☐NAF
  - Penis/ Testicles/ Vulva:_____ ☐NAF
  - Superficial inguinal lnn. [normally absent]:_____ ☐NAF

- Pelvic limb:_____ ☐NAF
  - Foot pads:_____ ☐NAF
  - Knuckling:_____ ☐NAF
  - Popliteal lnn.: ☐Enlarged Lt., ☐Enlarged Rt.,_____ ☐NAF

- Skin:_____ ☐NAF
- Tail:_____ ☐NAF
- Rectal☞☉:_____ ☐NAF

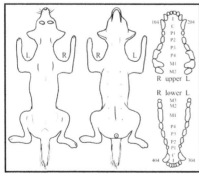
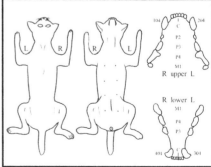

Problems List:

• **Problem #1**:

• **Problem #2**:

• **Problem #3**:

• **Problem #4**:

• **Problem #5**:

Diagnostic Plan	Treatment Plan

Case No._____

Patient	Age	Sex	Breed	Weight
	DOB:	Mn / Mi Fs / Fi	Color:	kg

Owner	Primary Veterinarian	Admit Date/ Time
Name: Phone:	Name: Phone:	Date: Time: AM / PM

• **Presenting Complaint**:_____

_____

_____

• **Medical Hx**:_____

_____

_____

• **When/ where obtained**: Date:_____; □Breeder, □Shelter, Other:_____

Drug/ Suppl.	Amount	Dose (mg/kg)	Route	Frequency	Date Started

• **Vaccine status – Dog**: □Rab □Parv □Dist □Aden; □Para □Lep □Bord □Influ □Lyme
• **Vaccine status – Cat**: □Rab □Herp □Cali □Pan □FeLV[kittens]; □FIV □Chlam □Bord
• **Heartworm / Flea & Tick / Intestinal Parasites**:
  ◦ *Last Heartworm Test*: Date:_____, □IDK; Test Results: □Pos, □Neg, □IDK
  ◦ *Monthly heartworm preventative*: □no □yes, Product:_____
  ◦ *Monthly flea & tick preventative*: □no □yes, Product:_____
  ◦ *Monthly dewormer*: □no □yes, Product:_____
• **Surgical Hx**: □Spay/Neuter; Date:_____; Other:_____
• **Environment**: □Indoor, □Outdoor, Time spent outdoors/ Other:_____
• **Housemates**: Dogs:_____ Cats:_____ Other:_____
• **Diet**: □Wet, □Dry; Brand/ Amt.:_____

Appetite	□Normal, □↑, □↓
Weight	□Normal, □↑, □↓; Past Wt.:_____ kg; Date:_____; Δ:_____
Thirst	□Normal, □↑, □↓
Urination	□Normal, □↑, □↓, □Blood, □Strain
Defecation	□Normal, □↑, □↓, □Blood, □Strain, □Diarrhea, □Mucus
Discharge	□No, □Yes; Onset/ Describe:
Cough/ Sneeze	□No, □Yes; Onset/ Describe:
Vomit	□No, □Yes; Onset/ Describe:
Respiration	□Normal, □↑ Rate, □↑ Effort
Energy level	□Normal, □Lethargic, □Exercise intolerance

• **Travel Hx**: □None, Other:_____
• **Exposure to**: □Standing water, □Wildlife, □Board/daycare, □Dog park, □Groomer
• **Adverse reactions to food/ meds**: □None, Other:_____
• **Can give oral meds**: □no □yes; Helpful Tricks:_____

Physical Exam – General:

- **Body Weight**:_____kg   **Body Condition Score**:_____/9

- **Temperature**:_____°F [*Dog-RI*: 100.9–102.4; *Cat-RI*: 98.1–102.1]

- **Heart**:
    - *Rate*:_____beats/min [Dog-RI: 60–180; Cat-RI: 140–240 (in hospital)]
    - *Rhythm*:   □Regular, □Irregular
    - *Sounds*:   □None, □Split sound, □Gallop, □Murmur, □Muffled
        - *Grade*:   □1–2[soft, only at PMI],   □3–4[moderate, mild radiate],   □5–6[strong radiate, thrill]
        - *Timing*: □Systolic, □Diastolic, □Continuous
        - *PMI*:

	PMI	Over	Anatomic Boundaries
□	Lt. apex	Mitral valve	5th to 6th ICS at level of CCJ
□	Lt. base	Ao + Pul outflow	2nd to 4th ICS above the CCJ
□	Rt. midheart	Tricuspid valve	3rd to 5th ICS near the CCJ
□	Rt. sternal border	Right ventricle	5th to 7th ICS immediately dorsal to the sternum
□	Sternal (cat)	Sternum	In cats, PMI offers very little clinical significance.

- *Vertebral Heart Size*: Dog = 8.7–10.5; Cat = 6.9–8.1 (from cranial edge of T4)
- *Innocent Murmur*: Grade 1-2, systolic, left base location, disappear by ~4 months of age, absent clinical signs

- **Pulses**:
    - *Pulse rate*:_____pulses/min
    - *Character*:   □Sync, □Async; □Normokinetic, □Hyper-, □Hypo-, □Variable

- **Lungs**:
    - *Respiratory rate*:_____breaths/min [*RI*: 16–30]
    - *Depth/Effort*: □Norm, □Pant, □Deep, □Shallow, □↑ Insp effort, □↑ Exp effort
    - *Sounds/Localization*:
        - □Norm BV, □Quiet BV, □Loud BV, □Crack, □Wheez, □Frict, □Muffled
        - □All fields, □Rt cran, □Rt mid, □Rt caud, □Lt cran, □Lt mid, □Lt caud
    - *Tracheal Auscultation/ Palpation*: □Normal, Other:_____

- **Pain Score**:_____ / 5   Localization:_____

- **Mentation**: □BAR   □Confused/   □Drowsy/   □Stuporous   □Coma
                 □QAR   Disoriented   Obtunded   (unresponsive
                 □Dull   unless aroused by
                                                           noxious stimuli)

- **Skin Elasticity**: □Normal skin turgor, □↓ Skin turgor, □Skin tent, □Gelatinous

- **Mucus Membranes**:
    - *CRT*:_____ [*RI*: 1–2; <1 = compensated shock, sepsis, heat stroke; <2 = acute decompensated shock; >2 = late decompensated shock, decreased cardiac output, hypothermia]
    - *Color*:_____ [*RI*: pink; red = compensated shock, sepsis, heat stroke; pale/white = anemia, shock; blue = cyanosis; yellow = hepatic disease, extravascular hemolysis; brown = met-Hb]
    - *Texture*:_____ [*RI*: moist = hydrated; tacky-to-dry = 5–12% dehydrated]

Physical Exam – Systems Checklist:

- Head:_____ ☐NAF
  - Ears: ☐Debris (mild / mod / sev) (AS / AD / AU), _____ ☐NAF
  - Eyes:_____ ☐NAF
    - Retinal:_____ ☐NAF

→ ⦿ Ⓛ		⦿ Ⓡ	
☐ Normal Direct	☐ Normal Indirect	☐ Normal Indirect	☐ Normal Direct
☐ Abnormal Direct	☐ Abnormal Indirect	☐ Abnormal Indirect	☐ Abnormal Direct

⦿ Ⓛ		⦿ Ⓡ ←	

  - Nose:_____ ☐NAF
  - Oral cavity: ☐Tarter/Gingivitis (mild / mod / sev), _____ ☐NAF
  - Mandibular lnn.: ☐Enlarged Lt., ☐Enlarged Rt., _____ ☐NAF

- Neck:_____ ☐NAF
  - Superficial cervical lnn.: ☐Enlarged Lt., ☐Enlarged Rt., ___ ☐NAF
  - Thyroid:_____ ☐NAF

- Thoracic limb:_____ ☐NAF
  - Foot pads:_____ ☐NAF
  - Knuckling:_____ ☐NAF
  - Axillary lnn. [normally absent]:_____ ☐NAF

- Thorax:_____ ☐NAF

- Abdomen:_____ ☐NAF
  - Mammary chain:_____ ☐NAF
  - Penis/ Testicles/ Vulva:_____ ☐NAF
  - Superficial inguinal lnn. [normally absent]:_____ ☐NAF

- Pelvic limb:_____ ☐NAF
  - Foot pads:_____ ☐NAF
  - Knuckling:_____ ☐NAF
  - Popliteal lnn.: ☐Enlarged Lt., ☐Enlarged Rt., _____ ☐NAF

- Skin:_____ ☐NAF
- Tail:_____ ☐NAF
- Rectal☞☉:_____ ☐NAF

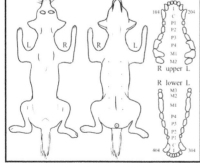
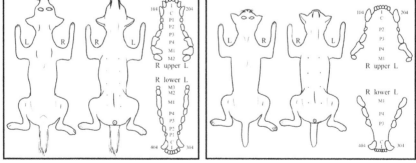

Problems List:

- **Problem #1**:

- **Problem #2**:

- **Problem #3**:

- **Problem #4**:

- **Problem #5**:

Diagnostic Plan	Treatment Plan

Case No._____

Patient		Age	Sex	Breed		Weight
	DOB:		Mn / Mi Fs / Fi	Color:		kg

Owner		Primary Veterinarian	Admit Date/ Time	
Name: Phone:		Name: Phone:	Date: Time:	AM / PM

• **Presenting Complaint**:_____

_____

• **Medical Hx**:_____

_____

• **When/ where obtained**: Date:_____; ☐Breeder, ☐Shelter, Other:_____

Drug/ Suppl.	Amount	Dose (mg/kg)	Route	Frequency	Date Started

• **Vaccine status – Dog**: ☐Rab ☐Parv ☐Dist ☐Aden; ☐Para ☐Lep ☐Bord ☐Influ ☐Lyme
• **Vaccine status – Cat**: ☐Rab ☐Herp ☐Cali ☐Pan ☐FeLV[kittens]; ☐FIV ☐Chlam ☐Bord
• **Heartworm / Flea & Tick / Intestinal Parasites**:
  ◦ *Last Heartworm Test*: Date:_____, ☐IDK; Test Results: ☐Pos, ☐Neg, ☐IDK
  ◦ *Monthly heartworm preventative*: ☐no ☐yes, Product:_____
  ◦ *Monthly flea & tick preventative*: ☐no ☐yes, Product:_____
  ◦ *Monthly dewormer*: ☐no ☐yes, Product:_____
• **Surgical Hx**: ☐Spay/Neuter; Date:_____; Other:_____
• **Environment**: ☐Indoor, ☐Outdoor, Time spent outdoors/ Other:_____
• **Housemates**: Dogs:_____ Cats:_____ Other:_____
• **Diet**: ☐Wet, ☐Dry; Brand/ Amt.:_____

Appetite	☐Normal, ☐↑, ☐↓
Weight	☐Normal, ☐↑, ☐↓; Past Wt.:_____ kg; Date:_____; Δ:_____
Thirst	☐Normal, ☐↑, ☐↓
Urination	☐Normal, ☐↑, ☐↓, ☐Blood, ☐Strain
Defecation	☐Normal, ☐↑, ☐↓, ☐Blood, ☐Strain, ☐Diarrhea, ☐Mucus
Discharge	☐No, ☐Yes; Onset/ Describe:
Cough/ Sneeze	☐No, ☐Yes; Onset/ Describe:
Vomit	☐No, ☐Yes; Onset/ Describe:
Respiration	☐Normal, ☐↑ Rate, ☐↑ Effort
Energy level	☐Normal, ☐Lethargic, ☐Exercise intolerance

• **Travel Hx**: ☐None, Other:_____
• **Exposure to**: ☐Standing water, ☐Wildlife, ☐Board/daycare, ☐Dog park, ☐Groomer
• **Adverse reactions to food/ meds**: ☐None, Other:_____
• **Can give oral meds**: ☐no ☐yes; Helpful Tricks:_____

Physical Exam – General:

- **Body Weight**: _____ kg   **Body Condition Score**: _____ /9

- **Temperature**: _____ °F *[Dog-RI:* 100.9–102.4; *Cat-RI:* 98.1–102.1]

- **Heart**:
  - *Rate*: _____ beats/min [Dog-RI: 60–180; Cat-RI: 140–240 (in hospital)]
  - *Rhythm*: ☐Regular, ☐Irregular
  - *Sounds*: ☐None, ☐Split sound, ☐Gallop, ☐Murmur, ☐Muffled
    - *Grade*: ☐1–2[soft, only at PMI], ☐3–4[moderate, mild radiate], ☐5–6[strong radiate, thrill]
    - *Timing*: ☐Systolic, ☐Diastolic, ☐Continuous
    - *PMI*:

	PMI	Over	Anatomic Boundaries
☐	Lt. apex	Mitral valve	5th to 6th ICS at level of CCJ
☐	Lt. base	Ao + Pul outflow	2nd to 4th ICS above the CCJ
☐	Rt. midheart	Tricuspid valve	3rd to 5th ICS near the CCJ
☐	Rt. sternal border	Right ventricle	5th to 7th ICS immediately dorsal to the sternum
☐	Sternal (cat)	Sternum	In cats, PMI offers very little clinical significance.

  - *Vertebral Heart Size*: Dog = 8.7–10.5; Cat = 6.9–8.1 (from cranial edge of T4)
  - *Innocent Murmur*: Grade 1-2, systolic, left base location, disappear by ~4 months of age, absent clinical signs

- **Pulses**:
  - *Pulse rate*: _____ pulses/min
  - *Character*: ☐Sync, ☐Async; ☐Normokinetic, ☐Hyper-, ☐Hypo-, ☐Variable

- **Lungs**:
  - *Respiratory rate*: _____ breaths/min [RI: 16–30]
  - *Depth/Effort*: ☐Norm, ☐Pant, ☐Deep, ☐Shallow, ☐↑ Insp effort, ☐↑ Exp effort
  - *Sounds/Localization*:
    - ☐Norm BV, ☐Quiet BV, ☐Loud BV, ☐Crack, ☐Wheez, ☐Frict, ☐Muffled
    - ☐All fields, ☐Rt cran, ☐Rt mid, ☐Rt caud, ☐Lt cran, ☐Lt mid, ☐Lt caud
  - *Tracheal Auscultation/ Palpation*: ☐Normal, Other: _____

- **Pain Score**: _____ / 5   Localization: _____

- **Mentation**: ☐BAR   ☐Confused/   ☐Drowsy/   ☐Stuporous   ☐Coma
                 ☐QAR   Disoriented   Obtunded   (unresponsive
                 ☐Dull   unless aroused by
                                                             noxious stimuli)

- **Skin Elasticity**: ☐Normal skin turgor, ☐↓ Skin turgor, ☐Skin tent, ☐Gelatinous

- **Mucus Membranes**:
  - *CRT*: _____ [RI: 1–2; <1 = compensated shock, sepsis, heat stroke; <2 = acute decompensated shock; >2 = late decompensated shock, decreased cardiac output, hypothermia]
  - *Color*: _____ [RI: pink; red = compensated shock, sepsis, heat stroke; pale/white = anemia, shock; blue = cyanosis; yellow = hepatic disease, extravascular hemolysis; brown = met-Hb]
  - *Texture*: _____ [RI: moist = hydrated; tacky-to-dry = 5–12% dehydrated]

Physical Exam – Systems Checklist:

- Head:_____ ☐NAF
  - ◦ Ears: ☐Debris (mild / mod / sev) (AS / AD / AU),_____ ☐NAF
  - ◦ Eyes:_____ ☐NAF
    - ▪ Retinal:_____ ☐NAF

→ Ⓛ		Ⓡ		Ⓛ		Ⓡ ←	
☐	Normal Direct	☐	Normal Indirect	☐	Normal Indirect	☐	Normal Direct
☐	Abnormal Direct	☐	Abnormal Indirect	☐	Abnormal Indirect	☐	Abnormal Direct

  - ◦ Nose:_____ ☐NAF
  - ◦ Oral cavity: ☐Tarter/Gingivitis (mild / mod / sev),_____ ☐NAF
  - ◦ Mandibular lnn.: ☐Enlarged Lt., ☐Enlarged Rt.,_____ ☐NAF

- Neck:_____ ☐NAF
  - ◦ Superficial cervical lnn.: ☐Enlarged Lt., ☐Enlarged Rt.,_____ ☐NAF
  - ◦ Thyroid:_____ ☐NAF

- Thoracic limb:_____ ☐NAF
  - ◦ Foot pads:_____ ☐NAF
  - ◦ Knuckling:_____ ☐NAF
  - ◦ Axillary lnn. [normally absent]:_____ ☐NAF

- Thorax:_____ ☐NAF

- Abdomen:_____ ☐NAF
  - ◦ Mammary chain:_____ ☐NAF
  - ◦ Penis/ Testicles/ Vulva:_____ ☐NAF
  - ◦ Superficial inguinal lnn. [normally absent]:_____ ☐NAF

- Pelvic limb:_____ ☐NAF
  - ◦ Foot pads:_____ ☐NAF
  - ◦ Knuckling:_____ ☐NAF
  - ◦ Popliteal lnn.: ☐Enlarged Lt., ☐Enlarged Rt.,_____ ☐NAF

- Skin:_____ ☐NAF
- Tail:_____ ☐NAF
- Rectal☞☉:_____ ☐NAF

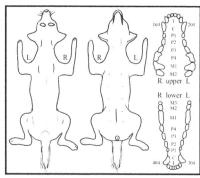

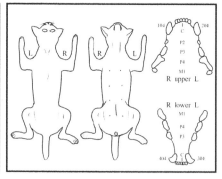

Problems List:

• **Problem #1**:

• **Problem #2**:

• **Problem #3**:

• **Problem #4**:

• **Problem #5**:

Diagnostic Plan	Treatment Plan

Case No._____

Patient	Age	Sex	Breed	Weight
	DOB:	Mn / Mi Fs / Fi	Color:	kg

Owner	Primary Veterinarian	Admit Date/ Time
Name: Phone:	Name: Phone:	Date: Time: AM / PM

• **Presenting Complaint**:_____
_____
_____

• **Medical Hx**:_____
_____
_____

• **When/ where obtained**:   Date:_____; ☐Breeder, ☐Shelter, Other:_____

Drug/ Suppl.	Amount	Dose (mg/kg)	Route	Frequency	Date Started

• **Vaccine status – Dog**: ☐Rab ☐Parv ☐Dist ☐Aden; ☐Para ☐Lep ☐Bord ☐Influ ☐Lyme
• **Vaccine status – Cat**: ☐Rab ☐Herp ☐Cali ☐Pan ☐FeLV[kittens]; ☐FIV ☐Chlam ☐Bord
• **Heartworm / Flea & Tick / Intestinal Parasites**:
  ◦ *Last Heartworm Test*: Date:_____, ☐IDK; Test Results: ☐Pos, ☐Neg, ☐IDK
  ◦ *Monthly heartworm preventative*:   ☐no ☐yes, Product:_____
  ◦ *Monthly flea & tick preventative*: ☐no ☐yes, Product:_____
  ◦ *Monthly dewormer*:   ☐no ☐yes, Product:_____
• **Surgical Hx**:   ☐Spay/Neuter; Date:_____; Other:_____
• **Environment**: ☐Indoor, ☐Outdoor, Time spent outdoors/ Other:_____
• **Housemates**: Dogs:_____ Cats:_____ Other:_____
• **Diet**: ☐Wet, ☐Dry; Brand/ Amt.:_____

Appetite	☐Normal, ☐↑, ☐↓
Weight	☐Normal, ☐↑, ☐↓; Past Wt.:_____ kg; Date:_____; Δ:_____
Thirst	☐Normal, ☐↑, ☐↓
Urination	☐Normal, ☐↑, ☐↓, ☐Blood, ☐Strain
Defecation	☐Normal, ☐↑, ☐↓, ☐Blood, ☐Strain, ☐Diarrhea, ☐Mucus
Discharge	☐No, ☐Yes; Onset/ Describe:
Cough/ Sneeze	☐No, ☐Yes; Onset/ Describe:
Vomit	☐No, ☐Yes; Onset/ Describe:
Respiration	☐Normal, ☐↑ Rate, ☐↑ Effort
Energy level	☐Normal, ☐Lethargic, ☐Exercise intolerance

• **Travel Hx**: ☐None, Other:_____
• **Exposure to**: ☐Standing water, ☐Wildlife, ☐Board/daycare, ☐Dog park, ☐Groomer
• **Adverse reactions to food/ meds**: ☐None, Other:_____
• **Can give oral meds**: ☐no ☐yes; Helpful Tricks:_____

Physical Exam – General:

- **Body Weight:**_____kg   **Body Condition Score:**____/9

- **Temperature:**_____°F [*Dog-RI*: 100.9–102.4; *Cat-RI*: 98.1–102.1]

- **Heart:**
  - *Rate*:_____beats/min [Dog-RI: 60–180; Cat-RI: 140–240 (in hospital)]
  - *Rhythm*: ☐Regular, ☐Irregular
  - *Sounds*: ☐None, ☐Split sound, ☐Gallop, ☐Murmur, ☐Muffled
    - *Grade*: ☐1–2[soft, only at PMI], ☐3–4[moderate, mild radiate], ☐5–6[strong radiate, thrill]
    - *Timing*: ☐Systolic, ☐Diastolic, ☐Continuous
    - *PMI*:

	PMI	Over	Anatomic Boundaries
☐	Lt. apex	Mitral valve	5th to 6th ICS at level of CCJ
☐	Lt. base	Ao + Pul outflow	2nd to 4th ICS above the CCJ
☐	Rt. midheart	Tricuspid valve	3rd to 5th ICS near the CCJ
☐	Rt. sternal border	Right ventricle	5th to 7th ICS immediately dorsal to the sternum
☐	Sternal (cat)	Sternum	In cats, PMI offers very little clinical significance.

  -     •   *Vertebral Heart Size*: Dog = 8.7–10.5; Cat = 6.9–8.1 (from cranial edge of T4)
  -     •   *Innocent Murmur*: Grade 1-2, systolic, left base location, disappear by ~4 months of age, absent clinical signs

- **Pulses:**
  - *Pulse rate*:_____pulses/min
  - *Character*: ☐Sync, ☐Async; ☐Normokinetic, ☐Hyper-, ☐Hypo-, ☐Variable

- **Lungs:**
  - *Respiratory rate*:_____breaths/min [*RI*: 16–30]
  - *Depth/Effort*: ☐Norm, ☐Pant, ☐Deep, ☐Shallow, ☐↑ Insp effort, ☐↑ Exp effort
  - *Sounds/Localization*:
    - ☐Norm BV, ☐Quiet BV, ☐Loud BV, ☐Crack, ☐Wheez, ☐Frict, ☐Muffled
    - ☐All fields, ☐Rt cran, ☐Rt mid, ☐Rt caud, ☐Lt cran, ☐Lt mid, ☐Lt caud
  - *Tracheal Auscultation/ Palpation*: ☐Normal, Other:_____

- **Pain Score:**_____ / 5   Localization:_____

- **Mentation:** ☐BAR   ☐Confused/   ☐Drowsy/   ☐Stuporous   ☐Coma
                 ☐QAR   Disoriented   Obtunded   (unresponsive
                 ☐Dull   unless aroused by
                                                      noxious stimuli)

- **Skin Elasticity:** ☐Normal skin turgor, ☐↓ Skin turgor, ☐Skin tent, ☐Gelatinous

- **Mucus Membranes:**
  - *CRT*:_____ [*RI*: 1–2; <1 = compensated shock, sepsis, heat stroke; <2 = acute decompensated shock; >2 = late decompensated shock, decreased cardiac output, hypothermia]
  - *Color*:_____ [*RI*: pink; red = compensated shock, sepsis, heat stroke; pale/white = anemia, shock; blue = cyanosis; yellow = hepatic disease, extravascular hemolysis; brown = met-Hb]
  - *Texture*:_____ [*RI*: moist = hydrated; tacky-to-dry = 5–12% dehydrated]

Physical Exam – Systems Checklist:

- Head: ____ ☐NAF
  - Ears: ☐Debris (mild / mod / sev) (AS / AD / AU), ______________________ ☐NAF
  - Eyes: ____ ☐NAF
    - Retinal: ____ ☐NAF

→ (L)		(R)		(L)		(R) ←	
☐	Normal Direct	☐	Normal Indirect	☐	Normal Indirect	☐	Normal Direct
☐	Abnormal Direct	☐	Abnormal Indirect	☐	Abnormal Indirect	☐	Abnormal Direct

  - Nose: ____ ☐NAF
  - Oral cavity: ☐Tarter/Gingivitis (mild / mod / sev), ______________________ ☐NAF
  - Mandibular lnn.: ☐Enlarged Lt., ☐Enlarged Rt., ______________________ ☐NAF

- Neck: ____ ☐NAF
  - Superficial cervical lnn.: ☐Enlarged Lt., ☐Enlarged Rt., ______________ ☐NAF
  - Thyroid: ____ ☐NAF

- Thoracic limb: ____ ☐NAF
  - Foot pads: ____ ☐NAF
  - Knuckling: ____ ☐NAF
  - Axillary lnn. [normally absent]: ______________________________ ☐NAF

- Thorax: ____ ☐NAF

- Abdomen: ____ ☐NAF
  - Mammary chain: ____ ☐NAF
  - Penis/ Testicles/ Vulva: ______________________________________ ☐NAF
  - Superficial inguinal lnn. [normally absent]: ______________________ ☐NAF

- Pelvic limb: ____ ☐NAF
  - Foot pads: ____ ☐NAF
  - Knuckling: ____ ☐NAF
  - Popliteal lnn.: ☐Enlarged Lt., ☐Enlarged Rt., ______________________ ☐NAF

- Skin: ____ ☐NAF
- Tail: ____ ☐NAF
- Rectal☞⊙: ____ ☐NAF

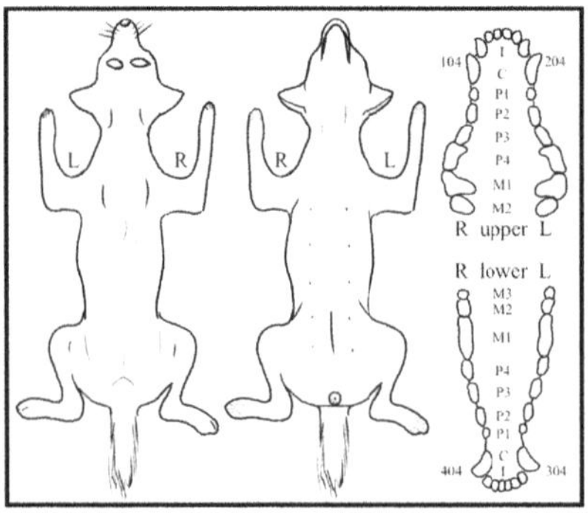

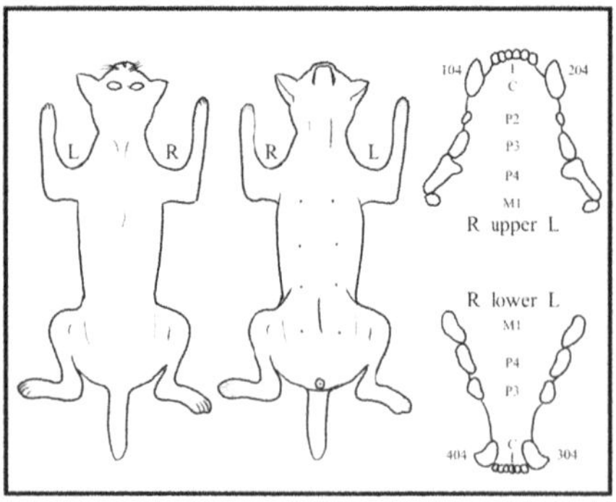

Problems List:

• **Problem #1**:

• **Problem #2**:

• **Problem #3**:

• **Problem #4**:

• **Problem #5**:

Diagnostic Plan	Treatment Plan

Case No._____

Patient		Age	Sex	Breed		Weight
		DOB:	Mn / Mi Fs / Fi	Color:		kg

Owner		Primary Veterinarian	Admit Date/ Time
Name: Phone:		Name: Phone:	Date: Time: AM / PM

• **Presenting Complaint**:_____

_____

• **Medical Hx**:_____

_____

• **When/ where obtained**:   Date:_____ ; □Breeder, □Shelter, Other:_____

Drug/ Suppl.	Amount	Dose (mg/kg)	Route	Frequency	Date Started

• **Vaccine status – Dog**: □Rab □Parv □Dist □Aden; □Para □Lep □Bord □Influ □Lyme
• **Vaccine status – Cat**: □Rab □Herp □Cali □Pan □FeLV[kittens]; □FIV □Chlam □Bord
• **Heartworm / Flea & Tick / Intestinal Parasites**:
   ◦ *Last Heartworm Test*: Date:_____, □IDK; Test Results: □Pos, □Neg, □IDK
   ◦ *Monthly heartworm preventative*:   □no □yes, Product:_____
   ◦ *Monthly flea & tick preventative*:   □no □yes, Product:_____
   ◦ *Monthly dewormer*:   □no □yes, Product:_____
• **Surgical Hx**: □Spay/Neuter; Date:_____ ; Other:_____
• **Environment**: □Indoor, □Outdoor, Time spent outdoors/ Other:_____
• **Housemates**: Dogs:_____ Cats:_____ Other:_____
• **Diet**: □Wet, □Dry; Brand/ Amt.:_____

Appetite	□Normal, □↑, □↓
Weight	□Normal, □↑, □↓; Past Wt.:_____ kg; Date:_____ ; Δ:_____
Thirst	□Normal, □↑, □↓
Urination	□Normal, □↑, □↓, □Blood, □Strain
Defecation	□Normal, □↑, □↓, □Blood, □Strain, □Diarrhea, □Mucus
Discharge	□No, □Yes; Onset/ Describe:
Cough/ Sneeze	□No, □Yes; Onset/ Describe:
Vomit	□No, □Yes; Onset/ Describe:
Respiration	□Normal, □↑ Rate, □↑ Effort
Energy level	□Normal, □Lethargic, □Exercise intolerance

• **Travel Hx**: □None, Other:_____
• **Exposure to**: □Standing water, □Wildlife, □Board/daycare, □Dog park, □Groomer
• **Adverse reactions to food/ meds**: □None, Other:_____
• **Can give oral meds**: □no □yes; Helpful Tricks:_____

Physical Exam – General:

- **Body Weight**:_____kg   **Body Condition Score**:_____/9

- **Temperature**:_____°F [Dog-RI: 100.9–102.4; Cat-RI: 98.1–102.1]

- **Heart**:
  - Rate:_____beats/min [Dog-RI: 60–180; Cat-RI: 140–240 (in hospital)]
  - Rhythm: □Regular, □Irregular
  - Sounds: □None, □Split sound, □Gallop, □Murmur, □Muffled
    - Grade: □1–2[soft, only at PMI], □3–4[moderate, mild radiate], □5–6[strong radiate, thrill]
    - Timing: □Systolic, □Diastolic, □Continuous
    - PMI:

	PMI	Over	Anatomic Boundaries
□	Lt. apex	Mitral valve	5th to 6th ICS at level of CCJ
□	Lt. base	Ao + Pul outflow	2nd to 4th ICS above the CCJ
□	Rt. midheart	Tricuspid valve	3rd to 5th ICS near the CCJ
□	Rt. sternal border	Right ventricle	5th to 7th ICS immediately dorsal to the sternum
□	Sternal (cat)	Sternum	In cats, PMI offers very little clinical significance.

  - • Vertebral Heart Size: Dog = 8.7–10.5; Cat = 6.9–8.1 (from cranial edge of T4)
  - • Innocent Murmur: Grade 1-2, systolic, left base location, disappear by ~4 months of age, absent clinical signs

- **Pulses**:
  - Pulse rate:_____pulses/min
  - Character: □Sync, □Async; □Normokinetic, □Hyper-, □Hypo-, □Variable

- **Lungs**:
  - Respiratory rate:_____breaths/min [RI: 16–30]
  - Depth/Effort: □Norm, □Pant, □Deep, □Shallow, □↑ Insp effort, □↑ Exp effort
  - Sounds/Localization:
    - □Norm BV, □Quiet BV, □Loud BV, □Crack, □Wheez, □Frict, □Muffled
    - □All fields, □Rt cran, □Rt mid, □Rt caud, □Lt cran, □Lt mid, □Lt caud
  - Tracheal Auscultation/ Palpation: □Normal, Other:_____

- **Pain Score**:_____ / 5   Localization:_____

- **Mentation**: □BAR   □Confused/   □Drowsy/   □Stuporous   □Coma
                  □QAR   Disoriented   Obtunded   (unresponsive
                  □Dull   unless aroused by
                                                       noxious stimuli)

- **Skin Elasticity**: □Normal skin turgor, □↓ Skin turgor, □Skin tent, □Gelatinous

- **Mucus Membranes**:
  - CRT:_____ [RI: 1–2; <1 = compensated shock, sepsis, heat stroke; <2 = acute decompensated shock; >2 = late decompensated shock, decreased cardiac output, hypothermia]
  - Color:_____ [RI: pink; red = compensated shock, sepsis, heat stroke; pale/white = anemia, shock; blue = cyanosis; yellow = hepatic disease, extravascular hemolysis; brown = met-Hb]
  - Texture:_____ [RI: moist = hydrated; tacky-to-dry = 5–12% dehydrated]

Physical Exam – Systems Checklist:

- Head:_____ ☐NAF
  - Ears: ☐Debris (mild / mod / sev) (AS / AD / AU), _____ ☐NAF
  - Eyes:_____ ☐NAF
    - Retinal:_____ ☐NAF

→ Ⓛ	Ⓡ	Ⓛ	Ⓡ ←
☐ Normal Direct	☐ Normal Indirect	☐ Normal Indirect	☐ Normal Direct
☐ Abnormal Direct	☐ Abnormal Indirect	☐ Abnormal Indirect	☐ Abnormal Direct

  - Nose:_____ ☐NAF
  - Oral cavity: ☐Tarter/Gingivitis (mild / mod / sev), _____ ☐NAF
  - Mandibular lnn.: ☐Enlarged Lt., ☐Enlarged Rt., _____ ☐NAF

- Neck:_____ ☐NAF
  - Superficial cervical lnn.: ☐Enlarged Lt., ☐Enlarged Rt., ____ ☐NAF
  - Thyroid:_____ ☐NAF

- Thoracic limb:_____ ☐NAF
  - Foot pads:_____ ☐NAF
  - Knuckling:_____ ☐NAF
  - Axillary lnn. [normally absent]:_____ ☐NAF

- Thorax:_____ ☐NAF

- Abdomen:_____ ☐NAF
  - Mammary chain:_____ ☐NAF
  - Penis/ Testicles/ Vulva:_____ ☐NAF
  - Superficial inguinal lnn. [normally absent]:_____ ☐NAF

- Pelvic limb:_____ ☐NAF
  - Foot pads:_____ ☐NAF
  - Knuckling:_____ ☐NAF
  - Popliteal lnn.: ☐Enlarged Lt., ☐Enlarged Rt., _____ ☐NAF

- Skin:_____ ☐NAF
- Tail:_____ ☐NAF
- Rectal☞⊙:_____ ☐NAF

Problems List:

• **Problem #1**:

• **Problem #2**:

• **Problem #3**:

• **Problem #4**:

• **Problem #5**:

Diagnostic Plan	Treatment Plan

Case No._____

Patient	Age	Sex	Breed		Weight
	DOB:	Mn / Mi Fs / Fi	Color:		kg

Owner	Primary Veterinarian	Admit Date/ Time
Name: Phone:	Name: Phone:	Date: Time: AM / PM

• **Presenting Complaint**:_____
_____
_____

• **Medical Hx**:_____
_____
_____

• **When/ where obtained**: Date:_____; □Breeder, □Shelter, Other:_____

Drug/ Suppl.	Amount	Dose (mg/kg)	Route	Frequency	Date Started

• **Vaccine status – Dog**: □Rab □Parv □Dist □Aden; □Para □Lep □Bord □Influ □Lyme
• **Vaccine status – Cat**: □Rab □Herp □Cali □Pan □FeLV[kittens]; □FIV □Chlam □Bord
• **Heartworm / Flea & Tick / Intestinal Parasites**:
  ◦ *Last Heartworm Test*: Date:_____, □IDK; Test Results: □Pos, □Neg, □IDK
  ◦ *Monthly heartworm preventative*: □no □yes, Product:_____
  ◦ *Monthly flea & tick preventative*: □no □yes, Product:_____
  ◦ *Monthly dewormer*: □no □yes, Product:_____
• **Surgical Hx**: □Spay/Neuter; Date:_____; Other:_____
• **Environment**: □Indoor, □Outdoor, Time spent outdoors/ Other:_____
• **Housemates**: Dogs:_____ Cats:_____ Other:_____
• **Diet**: □Wet, □Dry; Brand/ Amt.:_____

Appetite	□Normal, □↑, □↓
Weight	□Normal, □↑, □↓; Past Wt.:_____ kg; Date:_____; Δ:_____
Thirst	□Normal, □↑, □↓
Urination	□Normal, □↑, □↓, □Blood, □Strain
Defecation	□Normal, □↑, □↓, □Blood, □Strain, □Diarrhea, □Mucus
Discharge	□No, □Yes; Onset/ Describe:
Cough/ Sneeze	□No, □Yes; Onset/ Describe:
Vomit	□No, □Yes; Onset/ Describe:
Respiration	□Normal, □↑ Rate, □↑ Effort
Energy level	□Normal, □Lethargic, □Exercise intolerance

• **Travel Hx**: □None, Other:_____
• **Exposure to**: □Standing water, □Wildlife, □Board/daycare, □Dog park, □Groomer
• **Adverse reactions to food/ meds**: □None, Other:_____
• **Can give oral meds**: □no □yes; Helpful Tricks:_____

Physical Exam – General:

- **Body Weight**:_____ kg   **Body Condition Score**:_____ /9

- **Temperature**:_____ °F [*Dog-RI*: 100.9–102.4; *Cat-RI*: 98.1–102.1]

- **Heart**:
  - *Rate*:_____ beats/min [Dog-RI: 60–180; Cat-RI: 140–240 (in hospital)]
  - *Rhythm*:   ☐Regular, ☐Irregular
  - *Sounds*:   ☐None, ☐Split sound, ☐Gallop, ☐Murmur, ☐Muffled
    - *Grade*:   ☐1–2[soft, only at PMI], ☐3–4[moderate, mild radiate],   ☐5–6[strong radiate, thrill]
    - *Timing*: ☐Systolic, ☐Diastolic, ☐Continuous
    - *PMI*:

	PMI	Over	Anatomic Boundaries
☐	Lt. apex	Mitral valve	5th to 6th ICS at level of CCJ
☐	Lt. base	Ao + Pul outflow	2nd to 4th ICS above the CCJ
☐	Rt. midheart	Tricuspid valve	3rd to 5th ICS near the CCJ
☐	Rt. sternal border	Right ventricle	5th to 7th ICS immediately dorsal to the sternum
☐	Sternal (cat)	Sternum	In cats, PMI offers very little clinical significance.

- · *Vertebral Heart Size*: Dog = 8.7–10.5; Cat = 6.9–8.1 (from cranial edge of T4)
- · *Innocent Murmur*: Grade 1-2, systolic, left base location, disappear by ~4 months of age, absent clinical signs

- **Pulses**:
  - *Pulse rate*:_____ pulses/min
  - *Character*:   ☐Sync, ☐Async;   ☐Normokinetic, ☐Hyper-, ☐Hypo-, ☐Variable

- **Lungs**:
  - *Respiratory rate*:_____ breaths/min [*RI*: 16–30]
  - *Depth/Effort*: ☐Norm, ☐Pant, ☐Deep, ☐Shallow, ☐↑ Insp effort, ☐↑ Exp effort
  - *Sounds/Localization*:
    - ☐Norm BV, ☐Quiet BV, ☐Loud BV, ☐Crack, ☐Wheez, ☐Frict, ☐Muffled
    - ☐All fields, ☐Rt cran, ☐Rt mid, ☐Rt caud, ☐Lt cran, ☐Lt mid, ☐Lt caud
  - *Tracheal Auscultation/ Palpation*: ☐Normal, Other:_____

- **Pain Score**:_____ / 5   Localization:_____

- **Mentation**: ☐BAR   ☐Confused/   ☐Drowsy/   ☐Stuporous   ☐Coma
    ☐QAR   Disoriented   Obtunded   (unresponsive
    ☐Dull   unless aroused by
                                       noxious stimuli)

- **Skin Elasticity**: ☐Normal skin turgor, ☐↓ Skin turgor, ☐Skin tent, ☐Gelatinous

- **Mucus Membranes**:
  - *CRT*:_____ [*RI*: 1–2; <1 = compensated shock, sepsis, heat stroke; <2 = acute decompensated shock; >2 = late decompensated shock, decreased cardiac output, hypothermia]
  - *Color*:_____ [*RI*: pink; red = compensated shock, sepsis, heat stroke; pale/white = anemia, shock; blue = cyanosis; yellow = hepatic disease, extravascular hemolysis; brown = met-Hb]
  - *Texture*:_____ [*RI*: moist = hydrated; tacky-to-dry = 5–12% dehydrated]

Physical Exam – Systems Checklist:

- Head:_____ ☐NAF
  - ○ Ears: ☐Debris (mild / mod / sev) (AS / AD / AU),_____ ☐NAF
  - ○ Eyes:_____ ☐NAF
    - ▪ Retinal:_____ ☐NAF

→ ⦿ L		⦿ R		⦿ L		⦿ R ←	
☐	Normal Direct	☐	Normal Indirect	☐	Normal Indirect	☐	Normal Direct
☐	Abnormal Direct	☐	Abnormal Indirect	☐	Abnormal Indirect	☐	Abnormal Direct

  - ○ Nose:_____ ☐NAF
  - ○ Oral cavity: ☐Tarter/Gingivitis (mild / mod / sev),_____ ☐NAF
  - ○ Mandibular lnn.: ☐Enlarged Lt., ☐Enlarged Rt.,_____ ☐NAF

- Neck:_____ ☐NAF
  - ○ Superficial cervical lnn.: ☐Enlarged Lt., ☐Enlarged Rt.,_____ ☐NAF
  - ○ Thyroid:_____ ☐NAF

- Thoracic limb:_____ ☐NAF
  - ○ Foot pads:_____ ☐NAF
  - ○ Knuckling:_____ ☐NAF
  - ○ Axillary lnn. [normally absent]:_____ ☐NAF

- Thorax:_____ ☐NAF

- Abdomen:_____ ☐NAF
  - ○ Mammary chain:_____ ☐NAF
  - ○ Penis/ Testicles/ Vulva:_____ ☐NAF
  - ○ Superficial inguinal lnn. [normally absent]:_____ ☐NAF

- Pelvic limb:_____ ☐NAF
  - ○ Foot pads:_____ ☐NAF
  - ○ Knuckling:_____ ☐NAF
  - ○ Popliteal lnn.: ☐Enlarged Lt., ☐Enlarged Rt.,_____ ☐NAF

- Skin:_____ ☐NAF
- Tail:_____ ☐NAF
- Rectal☞⊙:_____ ☐NAF

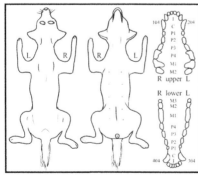
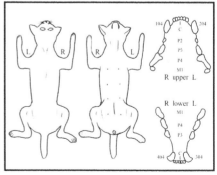

Problems List:

• **Problem #1**:

• **Problem #2**:

• **Problem #3**:

• **Problem #4**:

• **Problem #5**:

Diagnostic Plan	Treatment Plan

Case No._____

Patient	Age	Sex	Breed	Weight
	DOB:	Mn / Mi Fs / Fi	Color:	kg

Owner		Primary Veterinarian	Admit Date/ Time
Name: Phone:		Name: Phone:	Date: Time: AM / PM

• **Presenting Complaint**:_____
_____
_____

• **Medical Hx**:_____
_____
_____

• **When/ where obtained**:   Date:_____; ☐Breeder, ☐Shelter, Other:_____

Drug/ Suppl.	Amount	Dose (mg/kg)	Route	Frequency	Date Started

• **Vaccine status – Dog**: ☐Rab ☐Parv ☐Dist ☐Aden; ☐Para ☐Lep ☐Bord ☐Influ ☐Lyme
• **Vaccine status – Cat**: ☐Rab ☐Herp ☐Cali ☐Pan ☐FeLV[kittens]; ☐FIV ☐Chlam ☐Bord
• **Heartworm / Flea & Tick / Intestinal Parasites**:
  ◦ *Last Heartworm Test*: Date:_____, ☐IDK; Test Results: ☐Pos, ☐Neg, ☐IDK
  ◦ *Monthly heartworm preventative*:   ☐no ☐yes, Product:_____
  ◦ *Monthly flea & tick preventative*:   ☐no ☐yes, Product:_____
  ◦ *Monthly dewormer*:   ☐no ☐yes, Product:_____
• **Surgical Hx**:   ☐Spay/Neuter; Date:_____; Other:_____
• **Environment**: ☐Indoor, ☐Outdoor, Time spent outdoors/ Other:_____
• **Housemates**: Dogs:_____ Cats:_____ Other:_____
• **Diet**: ☐Wet, ☐Dry; Brand/ Amt.:_____

Appetite	☐Normal, ☐↑, ☐↓
Weight	☐Normal, ☐↑, ☐↓; Past Wt.:_____ kg; Date:_____; Δ:_____
Thirst	☐Normal, ☐↑, ☐↓
Urination	☐Normal, ☐↑, ☐↓, ☐Blood, ☐Strain
Defecation	☐Normal, ☐↑, ☐↓, ☐Blood, ☐Strain, ☐Diarrhea, ☐Mucus
Discharge	☐No, ☐Yes; Onset/ Describe:
Cough/ Sneeze	☐No, ☐Yes; Onset/ Describe:
Vomit	☐No, ☐Yes; Onset/ Describe:
Respiration	☐Normal, ☐↑ Rate, ☐↑ Effort
Energy level	☐Normal, ☐Lethargic, ☐Exercise intolerance

• **Travel Hx**: ☐None, Other:_____
• **Exposure to**: ☐Standing water, ☐Wildlife, ☐Board/daycare, ☐Dog park, ☐Groomer
• **Adverse reactions to food/ meds**: ☐None, Other:_____
• **Can give oral meds**: ☐no ☐yes; Helpful Tricks:_____

Physical Exam – General:

- **Body Weight**:_____kg   **Body Condition Score**:_____/9

- **Temperature**:_____°F [*Dog-RI*: 100.9–102.4; *Cat-RI*: 98.1–102.1]

- **Heart**:
  - *Rate*:_____beats/min [Dog-RI: 60–180; Cat-RI: 140–240 (in hospital)]
  - *Rhythm*:   □Regular, □Irregular
  - *Sounds*:   □None, □Split sound, □Gallop, □Murmur, □Muffled
    - *Grade*:   □1–2[soft, only at PMI], □3–4[moderate, mild radiate], □5–6[strong radiate, thrill]
    - *Timing*: □Systolic, □Diastolic, □Continuous
    - *PMI*:

	PMI	Over	Anatomic Boundaries
□	Lt. apex	Mitral valve	5th to 6th ICS at level of CCJ
□	Lt. base	Ao + Pul outflow	2nd to 4th ICS above the CCJ
□	Rt. midheart	Tricuspid valve	3rd to 5th ICS near the CCJ
□	Rt. sternal border	Right ventricle	5th to 7th ICS immediately dorsal to the sternum
□	Sternal (cat)	Sternum	In cats, PMI offers very little clinical significance.

  - • *Vertebral Heart Size*: Dog = 8.7–10.5; Cat = 6.9–8.1 (from cranial edge of T4)
  - • *Innocent Murmur*: Grade 1-2, systolic, left base location, disappear by ~4 months of age, absent clinical signs

- **Pulses**:
  - *Pulse rate*:_____pulses/min
  - *Character*:   □Sync, □Async; □Normokinetic, □Hyper-, □Hypo-, □Variable

- **Lungs**:
  - *Respiratory rate*:_____breaths/min [*RI*: 16–30]
  - *Depth/Effort*: □Norm, □Pant, □Deep, □Shallow, □↑ Insp effort, □↑ Exp effort
  - *Sounds/Localization*:
    - □Norm BV, □Quiet BV, □Loud BV, □Crack, □Wheez, □Frict, □Muffled
    - □All fields, □Rt cran, □Rt mid, □Rt caud, □Lt cran, □Lt mid, □Lt caud
  - *Tracheal Auscultation/ Palpation*: □Normal, Other:_____

- **Pain Score**:_____ / 5   Localization:_____

- **Mentation**: □BAR   □Confused/   □Drowsy/   □Stuporous   □Coma
                  □QAR   Disoriented   Obtunded   (unresponsive
                  □Dull   unless aroused by
                                                                  noxious stimuli)

- **Skin Elasticity**: □Normal skin turgor, □↓ Skin turgor, □Skin tent, □Gelatinous

- **Mucus Membranes**:
  - *CRT*:_____ [*RI*: 1–2; <1 = compensated shock, sepsis, heat stroke; <2 = acute decompensated shock; >2 = late decompensated shock, decreased cardiac output, hypothermia]
  - *Color*:_____ [*RI*: pink; red = compensated shock, sepsis, heat stroke; pale/white = anemia, shock; blue = cyanosis; yellow = hepatic disease, extravascular hemolysis; brown = met-Hb]
  - *Texture*:_____ [*RI*: moist = hydrated; tacky-to-dry = 5–12% dehydrated]

Physical Exam – Systems Checklist:

- Head:_____ ☐NAF
  - Ears: ☐Debris (mild / mod / sev) (AS / AD / AU),_____ ☐NAF
  - Eyes:_____ ☐NAF
    - Retinal:_____ ☐NAF

➡ Ⓛ	Ⓡ	Ⓛ	Ⓡ ⬅
☐ Normal Direct	☐ Normal Indirect	☐ Normal Indirect	☐ Normal Direct
☐ Abnormal Direct	☐ Abnormal Indirect	☐ Abnormal Indirect	☐ Abnormal Direct

  - Nose:_____ ☐NAF
  - Oral cavity: ☐Tarter/Gingivitis (mild / mod / sev),_____ ☐NAF
  - Mandibular lnn.: ☐Enlarged Lt., ☐Enlarged Rt.,_____ ☐NAF

- Neck:_____ ☐NAF
  - Superficial cervical lnn.: ☐Enlarged Lt., ☐Enlarged Rt.,_____ ☐NAF
  - Thyroid:_____ ☐NAF

- Thoracic limb:_____ ☐NAF
  - Foot pads:_____ ☐NAF
  - Knuckling:_____ ☐NAF
  - Axillary lnn. [normally absent]:_____ ☐NAF

- Thorax:_____ ☐NAF

- Abdomen:_____ ☐NAF
  - Mammary chain:_____ ☐NAF
  - Penis/ Testicles/ Vulva:_____ ☐NAF
  - Superficial inguinal lnn. [normally absent]:_____ ☐NAF

- Pelvic limb:_____ ☐NAF
  - Foot pads:_____ ☐NAF
  - Knuckling:_____ ☐NAF
  - Popliteal lnn.: ☐Enlarged Lt., ☐Enlarged Rt.,_____ ☐NAF

- Skin:_____ ☐NAF
- Tail:_____ ☐NAF
- Rectal☞☉:_____ ☐NAF

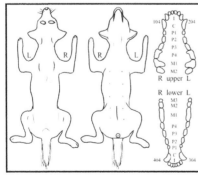

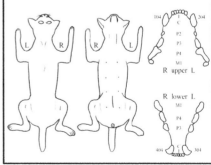

Problems List:

• Problem #1:

• Problem #2:

• Problem #3:

• Problem #4:

• Problem #5:

Diagnostic Plan	Treatment Plan

Case No._____

Patient	Age	Sex	Breed	Weight
	DOB:	Mn / Mi Fs / Fi	Color:	kg

Owner	Primary Veterinarian	Admit Date/ Time
Name: Phone:	Name: Phone:	Date: Time: AM / PM

• **Presenting Complaint**:_____
_____
_____

• **Medical Hx**:_____
_____
_____

• **When/ where obtained**:   Date:_____ ;   □Breeder, □Shelter, Other:_____

Drug/ Suppl.	Amount	Dose (mg/kg)	Route	Frequency	Date Started

• **Vaccine status – Dog**: □Rab □Parv □Dist □Aden; □Para □Lep □Bord □Influ □Lyme
• **Vaccine status – Cat**: □Rab □Herp □Cali □Pan □FeLV[kittens]; □FIV □Chlam □Bord
• **Heartworm / Flea & Tick / Intestinal Parasites**:
  ◦ *Last Heartworm Test*: Date:_____, □IDK; Test Results: □Pos, □Neg, □IDK
  ◦ *Monthly heartworm preventative*:   □no □yes, Product:_____
  ◦ *Monthly flea & tick preventative*:   □no □yes, Product:_____
  ◦ *Monthly dewormer*:   □no □yes, Product:_____
• **Surgical Hx**:   □Spay/Neuter; Date:_____ ;   Other:_____
• **Environment**: □Indoor, □Outdoor, Time spent outdoors/ Other:_____
• **Housemates**: Dogs:_____ Cats:_____ Other:_____
• **Diet**: □Wet, □Dry; Brand/ Amt.:_____

Appetite	□Normal, □↑, □↓
Weight	□Normal, □↑, □↓; Past Wt.:_____ kg; Date:_____ ; Δ:_____
Thirst	□Normal, □↑, □↓
Urination	□Normal, □↑, □↓, □Blood, □Strain
Defecation	□Normal, □↑, □↓, □Blood, □Strain, □Diarrhea, □Mucus
Discharge	□No, □Yes; Onset/ Describe:
Cough/ Sneeze	□No, □Yes; Onset/ Describe:
Vomit	□No, □Yes; Onset/ Describe:
Respiration	□Normal, □↑ Rate, □↑ Effort
Energy level	□Normal, □Lethargic, □Exercise intolerance

• **Travel Hx**: □None, Other:_____
• **Exposure to**: □Standing water, □Wildlife, □Board/daycare, □Dog park, □Groomer
• **Adverse reactions to food/ meds**: □None, Other:_____
• **Can give oral meds**: □no □yes; Helpful Tricks:_____

Physical Exam – General:

- **Body Weight**:_____kg   **Body Condition Score**:_____/9

- **Temperature**:_____°F [*Dog-RI*: 100.9–102.4; *Cat-RI*: 98.1–102.1]

- **Heart**:
  - *Rate*:_____beats/min [Dog-RI: 60–180; Cat-RI: 140–240 (in hospital)]
  - *Rhythm*:   □Regular, □Irregular
  - *Sounds*:   □None, □Split sound, □Gallop, □Murmur, □Muffled
    - *Grade*:   □1–2[soft, only at PMI], □3–4[moderate, mild radiate], □5–6[strong radiate, thrill]
    - *Timing*: □Systolic, □Diastolic, □Continuous
    - *PMI*:

	PMI	Over	Anatomic Boundaries
□	Lt. apex	Mitral valve	5th to 6th ICS at level of CCJ
□	Lt. base	Ao + Pul outflow	2nd to 4th ICS above the CCJ
□	Rt. midheart	Tricuspid valve	3rd to 5th ICS near the CCJ
□	Rt. sternal border	Right ventricle	5th to 7th ICS immediately dorsal to the sternum
□	Sternal (cat)	Sternum	In cats, PMI offers very little clinical significance.

- *Vertebral Heart Size*: Dog = 8.7–10.5; Cat = 6.9–8.1 (from cranial edge of T4)
- *Innocent Murmur*: Grade 1-2, systolic, left base location, disappear by ~4 months of age, absent clinical signs

- **Pulses**:
  - *Pulse rate*:_____pulses/min
  - *Character*:   □Sync, □Async;   □Normokinetic, □Hyper-, □Hypo-, □Variable

- **Lungs**:
  - *Respiratory rate*:_____breaths/min [*RI*: 16–30]
  - *Depth/Effort*: □Norm, □Pant, □Deep, □Shallow, □↑ Insp effort, □↑ Exp effort
  - *Sounds/Localization*:
    - □Norm BV, □Quiet BV, □Loud BV, □Crack, □Wheez, □Frict, □Muffled
    - □All fields, □Rt cran, □Rt mid, □Rt caud, □Lt cran, □Lt mid, □Lt caud
  - *Tracheal Auscultation/ Palpation*: □Normal, Other:_____

- **Pain Score**:_____ / 5   Localization:_____

- **Mentation**: □BAR   □Confused/   □Drowsy/   □Stuporous   □Coma
                 □QAR   Disoriented   Obtunded   (unresponsive
                 □Dull   unless aroused by
                                                               noxious stimuli)

- **Skin Elasticity**: □Normal skin turgor, □↓ Skin turgor, □Skin tent, □Gelatinous

- **Mucus Membranes**:
  - *CRT*:_____ [*RI*: 1–2; <1 = compensated shock, sepsis, heat stroke; <2 = acute decompensated shock; >2 = late decompensated shock, decreased cardiac output, hypothermia]
  - *Color*:_____ [*RI*: pink; red = compensated shock, sepsis, heat stroke; pale/white = anemia, shock; blue = cyanosis; yellow = hepatic disease, extravascular hemolysis; brown = met-Hb]
  - *Texture*:_____ [*RI*: moist = hydrated; tacky-to-dry = 5–12% dehydrated]

Physical Exam – Systems Checklist:

- Head:_____ ☐NAF
  - Ears: ☐Debris (mild / mod / sev) (AS / AD / AU), _____ ☐NAF
  - Eyes:_____ ☐NAF
    - Retinal:_____ ☐NAF

	⟶ Ⓛ		Ⓡ		Ⓛ		Ⓡ ⟵
☐	Normal Direct	☐	Normal Indirect	☐	Normal Indirect	☐	Normal Direct
☐	Abnormal Direct	☐	Abnormal Indirect	☐	Abnormal Indirect	☐	Abnormal Direct

  - Nose:_____ ☐NAF
  - Oral cavity: ☐Tarter/Gingivitis (mild / mod / sev), _____ ☐NAF
  - Mandibular lnn.: ☐Enlarged Lt., ☐Enlarged Rt., _____ ☐NAF

- Neck:_____ ☐NAF
  - Superficial cervical lnn.: ☐Enlarged Lt., ☐Enlarged Rt., _____ ☐NAF
  - Thyroid:_____ ☐NAF

- Thoracic limb:_____ ☐NAF
  - Foot pads:_____ ☐NAF
  - Knuckling:_____ ☐NAF
  - Axillary lnn. [normally absent]:_____ ☐NAF

- Thorax:_____ ☐NAF

- Abdomen:_____ ☐NAF
  - Mammary chain:_____ ☐NAF
  - Penis/ Testicles/ Vulva:_____ ☐NAF
  - Superficial inguinal lnn. [normally absent]:_____ ☐NAF

- Pelvic limb:_____ ☐NAF
  - Foot pads:_____ ☐NAF
  - Knuckling:_____ ☐NAF
  - Popliteal lnn.: ☐Enlarged Lt., ☐Enlarged Rt., _____ ☐NAF

- Skin:_____ ☐NAF
- Tail:_____ ☐NAF
- Rectal☞☉:_____ ☐NAF

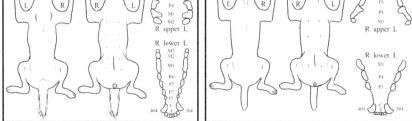

Problems List:

• Problem #1:

• Problem #2:

• Problem #3:

• Problem #4:

• Problem #5:

Diagnostic Plan	Treatment Plan

Case No._____

Patient	Age	Sex	Breed	Weight
	DOB:	Mn / Mi Fs / Fi	Color:	kg

Owner	Primary Veterinarian	Admit Date/ Time
Name: Phone:	Name: Phone:	Date: Time: AM / PM

• **Presenting Complaint**:_____
_____
_____

• **Medical Hx**:_____
_____
_____

• **When/ where obtained**:   Date:_____; □Breeder, □Shelter, Other:_____

Drug/ Suppl.	Amount	Dose (mg/kg)	Route	Frequency	Date Started

• **Vaccine status – Dog**: □Rab □Parv □Dist □Aden; □Para □Lep □Bord □Influ □Lyme
• **Vaccine status – Cat**: □Rab □Herp □Cali □Pan □FeLV[kittens]; □FIV □Chlam □Bord
• **Heartworm / Flea & Tick / Intestinal Parasites**:
   ◦ *Last Heartworm Test*: Date:_____, □IDK; Test Results: □Pos, □Neg, □IDK
   ◦ *Monthly heartworm preventative*:   □no □yes, Product:_____
   ◦ *Monthly flea & tick preventative*:   □no □yes, Product:_____
   ◦ *Monthly dewormer*:   □no □yes, Product:_____
• **Surgical Hx**:   □Spay/Neuter; Date:_____; Other:_____
• **Environment**: □Indoor, □Outdoor, Time spent outdoors/ Other:_____
• **Housemates**: Dogs:_____ Cats:_____ Other:_____
• **Diet**: □Wet, □Dry; Brand/ Amt.:_____

Appetite	□Normal, □↑, □↓
Weight	□Normal, □↑, □↓; Past Wt.:_____ kg; Date:_____; Δ:_____
Thirst	□Normal, □↑, □↓
Urination	□Normal, □↑, □↓, □Blood, □Strain
Defecation	□Normal, □↑, □↓, □Blood, □Strain, □Diarrhea, □Mucus
Discharge	□No, □Yes; Onset/ Describe:
Cough/ Sneeze	□No, □Yes; Onset/ Describe:
Vomit	□No, □Yes; Onset/ Describe:
Respiration	□Normal, □↑ Rate, □↑ Effort
Energy level	□Normal, □Lethargic, □Exercise intolerance

• **Travel Hx**: □None, Other:_____
• **Exposure to**: □Standing water, □Wildlife, □Board/daycare, □Dog park, □Groomer
• **Adverse reactions to food/ meds**: □None, Other:_____
• **Can give oral meds**: □no □yes; Helpful Tricks:_____

Physical Exam – General:

- **Body Weight**:_____kg   **Body Condition Score**:_____/9

- **Temperature**:_____°F [*Dog-RI*: 100.9–102.4; *Cat-RI*: 98.1–102.1]

- **Heart**:
  - *Rate*:_____beats/min [Dog-RI: 60–180; Cat-RI: 140–240 (in hospital)]
  - *Rhythm*: ☐Regular, ☐Irregular
  - *Sounds*: ☐None, ☐Split sound, ☐Gallop, ☐Murmur, ☐Muffled
    - *Grade*: ☐1–2[soft, only at PMI], ☐3–4[moderate, mild radiate], ☐5–6[strong radiate, thrill]
    - *Timing*: ☐Systolic, ☐Diastolic, ☐Continuous
    - *PMI*:

	PMI	Over	Anatomic Boundaries
☐	Lt. apex	Mitral valve	5th to 6th ICS at level of CCJ
☐	Lt. base	Ao + Pul outflow	2nd to 4th ICS above the CCJ
☐	Rt. midheart	Tricuspid valve	3rd to 5th ICS near the CCJ
☐	Rt. sternal border	Right ventricle	5th to 7th ICS immediately dorsal to the sternum
☐	Sternal (cat)	Sternum	In cats, PMI offers very little clinical significance.

  - • *Vertebral Heart Size*: Dog = 8.7–10.5; Cat = 6.9–8.1 (from cranial edge of T4)
  - • *Innocent Murmur*: Grade 1-2, systolic, left base location, disappear by ~4 months of age, absent clinical signs

- **Pulses**:
  - *Pulse rate*:_____pulses/min
  - *Character*: ☐Sync, ☐Async; ☐Normokinetic, ☐Hyper-, ☐Hypo-, ☐Variable

- **Lungs**:
  - *Respiratory rate*:_____breaths/min [*RI*: 16–30]
  - *Depth/Effort*: ☐Norm, ☐Pant, ☐Deep, ☐Shallow, ☐↑ Insp effort, ☐↑ Exp effort
  - *Sounds/Localization*:
    - ☐Norm BV, ☐Quiet BV, ☐Loud BV, ☐Crack, ☐Wheez, ☐Frict, ☐Muffled
    - ☐All fields, ☐Rt cran, ☐Rt mid, ☐Rt caud, ☐Lt cran, ☐Lt mid, ☐Lt caud
  - *Tracheal Auscultation/ Palpation*: ☐Normal, Other:_____

- **Pain Score**:_____ / 5   Localization:_____

- **Mentation**: ☐BAR   ☐Confused/   ☐Drowsy/   ☐Stuporous   ☐Coma
               ☐QAR   Disoriented   Obtunded   (unresponsive
               ☐Dull   unless aroused by
                                                        noxious stimuli)

- **Skin Elasticity**: ☐Normal skin turgor, ☐↓ Skin turgor, ☐Skin tent, ☐Gelatinous

- **Mucus Membranes**:
  - *CRT*:_____ [*RI*: 1–2; <1 = compensated shock, sepsis, heat stroke; <2 = acute decompensated shock; >2 = late decompensated shock, decreased cardiac output, hypothermia]
  - *Color*:_____ [*RI*: pink; red = compensated shock, sepsis, heat stroke; pale/white = anemia, shock; blue = cyanosis; yellow = hepatic disease, extravascular hemolysis; brown = met-Hb]
  - *Texture*:_____ [*RI*: moist = hydrated; tacky-to-dry = 5–12% dehydrated]

Physical Exam – Systems Checklist:

- Head:_____ ☐NAF
  - Ears: ☐Debris (mild / mod / sev) (AS / AD / AU),_____ ☐NAF
  - Eyes:_____ ☐NAF
    - Retinal:_____ ☐NAF

☐	Normal Direct	☐	Normal Indirect	☐	Normal Indirect	☐	Normal Direct
☐	Abnormal Direct	☐	Abnormal Indirect	☐	Abnormal Indirect	☐	Abnormal Direct

  - Nose:_____ ☐NAF
  - Oral cavity: ☐Tarter/Gingivitis (mild / mod / sev),_____ ☐NAF
  - Mandibular lnn.: ☐Enlarged Lt., ☐Enlarged Rt.,_____ ☐NAF

- Neck:_____ ☐NAF
  - Superficial cervical lnn.: ☐Enlarged Lt., ☐Enlarged Rt.,_____ ☐NAF
  - Thyroid:_____ ☐NAF

- Thoracic limb:_____ ☐NAF
  - Foot pads:_____ ☐NAF
  - Knuckling:_____ ☐NAF
  - Axillary lnn. [normally absent]:_____ ☐NAF

- Thorax:_____ ☐NAF

- Abdomen:_____ ☐NAF
  - Mammary chain:_____ ☐NAF
  - Penis/ Testicles/ Vulva:_____ ☐NAF
  - Superficial inguinal lnn. [normally absent]:_____ ☐NAF

- Pelvic limb:_____ ☐NAF
  - Foot pads:_____ ☐NAF
  - Knuckling:_____ ☐NAF
  - Popliteal lnn.: ☐Enlarged Lt., ☐Enlarged Rt.,_____ ☐NAF

- Skin:_____ ☐NAF
- Tail:_____ ☐NAF
- Rectal☞ ☉:_____ ☐NAF

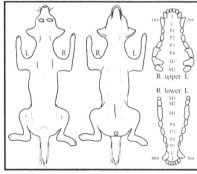
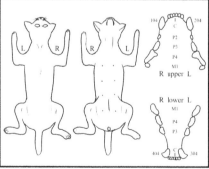

Problems List:

• Problem #1:

• Problem #2:

• Problem #3:

• Problem #4:

• Problem #5:

Diagnostic Plan	Treatment Plan

Case No._____

Patient	Age	Sex	Breed	Weight
	DOB:	Mn / Mi Fs / Fi	Color:	kg

Owner	Primary Veterinarian	Admit Date/ Time
Name: Phone:	Name: Phone:	Date: Time: AM / PM

• **Presenting Complaint**:_____

_____

• **Medical Hx**:_____

_____

• **When/ where obtained**: Date:_____ ; ☐Breeder, ☐Shelter, Other:_____

Drug/ Suppl.	Amount	Dose (mg/kg)	Route	Frequency	Date Started

• **Vaccine status – Dog**: ☐Rab ☐Parv ☐Dist ☐Aden; ☐Para ☐Lep ☐Bord ☐Influ ☐Lyme
• **Vaccine status – Cat**: ☐Rab ☐Herp ☐Cali ☐Pan ☐FeLV[kittens]; ☐FIV ☐Chlam ☐Bord
• **Heartworm / Flea & Tick / Intestinal Parasites**:
  ◦ *Last Heartworm Test*: Date:_____, ☐IDK; Test Results: ☐Pos, ☐Neg, ☐IDK
  ◦ *Monthly heartworm preventative*: ☐no ☐yes, Product:_____
  ◦ *Monthly flea & tick preventative*: ☐no ☐yes, Product:_____
  ◦ *Monthly dewormer*: ☐no ☐yes, Product:_____
• **Surgical Hx**: ☐Spay/Neuter; Date:_____; Other:_____
• **Environment**: ☐Indoor, ☐Outdoor, Time spent outdoors/ Other:_____
• **Housemates**: Dogs:____ Cats:____ Other:_____
• **Diet**: ☐Wet, ☐Dry; Brand/ Amt.:_____

Appetite	☐Normal, ☐↑, ☐↓
Weight	☐Normal, ☐↑, ☐↓; Past Wt.:_____ kg; Date:_____; Δ:_____
Thirst	☐Normal, ☐↑, ☐↓
Urination	☐Normal, ☐↑, ☐↓, ☐Blood, ☐Strain
Defecation	☐Normal, ☐↑, ☐↓, ☐Blood, ☐Strain, ☐Diarrhea, ☐Mucus
Discharge	☐No, ☐Yes; Onset/ Describe:
Cough/ Sneeze	☐No, ☐Yes; Onset/ Describe:
Vomit	☐No, ☐Yes; Onset/ Describe:
Respiration	☐Normal, ☐↑ Rate, ☐↑ Effort
Energy level	☐Normal, ☐Lethargic, ☐Exercise intolerance

• **Travel Hx**: ☐None, Other:_____
• **Exposure to**: ☐Standing water, ☐Wildlife, ☐Board/daycare, ☐Dog park, ☐Groomer
• **Adverse reactions to food/ meds**: ☐None, Other:_____
• **Can give oral meds**: ☐no ☐yes; Helpful Tricks:_____

<h1 style="text-align:center"><u>Physical Exam – General</u>:</h1>

• **Body Weight**:_____kg   **Body Condition Score**:_____/9

• **Temperature**:_____°F [*Dog-RI*: 100.9–102.4; *Cat-RI*: 98.1–102.1]

• **Heart**:
- ◦ *Rate*:_____beats/min [Dog-RI: 60–180; Cat-RI: 140–240 (in hospital)]
- ◦ *Rhythm*:   ☐Regular, ☐Irregular
- ◦ *Sounds*:   ☐None, ☐Split sound, ☐Gallop, ☐Murmur, ☐Muffled
  - ▪ *Grade*:   ☐1–2[soft, only at PMI], ☐3–4[moderate, mild radiate], ☐5–6[strong radiate, thrill]
  - ▪ *Timing*: ☐Systolic, ☐Diastolic, ☐Continuous
  - ▪ *PMI*:

	PMI	Over	Anatomic Boundaries
☐	Lt. apex	Mitral valve	5th to 6th ICS at level of CCJ
☐	Lt. base	Ao + Pul outflow	2nd to 4th ICS above the CCJ
☐	Rt. midheart	Tricuspid valve	3rd to 5th ICS near the CCJ
☐	Rt. sternal border	Right ventricle	5th to 7th ICS immediately dorsal to the sternum
☐	Sternal (cat)	Sternum	In cats, PMI offers very little clinical significance.

- • *Vertebral Heart Size*: Dog = 8.7–10.5; Cat = 6.9–8.1 (from cranial edge of T4)
- • *Innocent Murmur*: Grade 1-2, systolic, left base location, disappear by ~4 months of age, absent clinical signs

• **Pulses**:
- ◦ *Pulse rate*:_____pulses/min
- ◦ *Character*:   ☐Sync, ☐Async; ☐Normokinetic, ☐Hyper-, ☐Hypo-, ☐Variable

• **Lungs**:
- ◦ *Respiratory rate*:_____breaths/min [*RI*: 16–30]
- ◦ *Depth/Effort*: ☐Norm, ☐Pant, ☐Deep, ☐Shallow, ☐↑ Insp effort, ☐↑ Exp effort
- ◦ *Sounds/Localization*:
  - ▪ ☐Norm BV, ☐Quiet BV, ☐Loud BV, ☐Crack, ☐Wheez, ☐Frict, ☐Muffled
  - ▪ ☐All fields, ☐Rt cran, ☐Rt mid, ☐Rt caud, ☐Lt cran, ☐Lt mid, ☐Lt caud
- ◦ *Tracheal Auscultation/ Palpation*: ☐Normal, Other:_____

• **Pain Score**:_____ / 5   Localization:_____

• **Mentation**: ☐BAR   ☐Confused/   ☐Drowsy/   ☐Stuporous   ☐Coma
                ☐QAR   Disoriented   Obtunded   (unresponsive
                ☐Dull   unless aroused by
                                                    noxious stimuli)

• **Skin Elasticity**: ☐Normal skin turgor, ☐↓ Skin turgor, ☐Skin tent, ☐Gelatinous

• **Mucus Membranes**:
- ◦ *CRT*:_____ [*RI*: 1–2; <1 = compensated shock, sepsis, heat stroke; <2 = acute decompensated shock; >2 = late decompensated shock, decreased cardiac output, hypothermia]
- ◦ *Color*:_____ [*RI*: pink; red = compensated shock, sepsis, heat stroke; pale/white = anemia, shock; blue = cyanosis; yellow = hepatic disease, extravascular hemolysis; brown = met-Hb]
- ◦ *Texture*:_____ [*RI*: moist = hydrated; tacky-to-dry = 5–12% dehydrated]

Physical Exam – Systems Checklist:

- Head:_____ ☐NAF
  - Ears: ☐Debris (mild / mod / sev) (AS / AD / AU),_____ ☐NAF
  - Eyes:_____ ☐NAF
    - Retinal:_____ ☐NAF

→ Ⓛ		Ⓡ		Ⓛ		Ⓡ ←	
☐	Normal Direct	☐	Normal Indirect	☐	Normal Indirect	☐	Normal Direct
☐	Abnormal Direct	☐	Abnormal Indirect	☐	Abnormal Indirect	☐	Abnormal Direct

  - Nose:_____ ☐NAF
  - Oral cavity: ☐Tarter/Gingivitis (mild / mod / sev),_____ ☐NAF
  - Mandibular lnn.: ☐Enlarged Lt., ☐Enlarged Rt.,_____ ☐NAF

- Neck:_____ ☐NAF
  - Superficial cervical lnn.: ☐Enlarged Lt., ☐Enlarged Rt.,_____ ☐NAF
  - Thyroid:_____ ☐NAF

- Thoracic limb:_____ ☐NAF
  - Foot pads:_____ ☐NAF
  - Knuckling:_____ ☐NAF
  - Axillary lnn. [normally absent]:_____ ☐NAF

- Thorax:_____ ☐NAF

- Abdomen:_____ ☐NAF
  - Mammary chain:_____ ☐NAF
  - Penis/ Testicles/ Vulva:_____ ☐NAF
  - Superficial inguinal lnn. [normally absent]:_____ ☐NAF

- Pelvic limb:_____ ☐NAF
  - Foot pads:_____ ☐NAF
  - Knuckling:_____ ☐NAF
  - Popliteal lnn.: ☐Enlarged Lt., ☐Enlarged Rt.,_____ ☐NAF

- Skin:_____ ☐NAF
- Tail:_____ ☐NAF
- Rectal☞☉:_____ ☐NAF

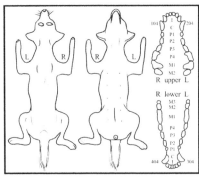
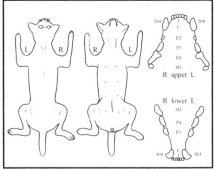

Problems List:

• Problem #1:

• Problem #2:

• Problem #3:

• Problem #4:

• Problem #5:

Diagnostic Plan	Treatment Plan

Patient	Age	Sex	Breed	Weight
	DOB:	Mn / Mi Fs / Fi	Color:	kg

Owner	Primary Veterinarian	Admit Date/ Time
Name: Phone:	Name: Phone:	Date: Time: AM / PM

• **Presenting Complaint**:_____

_____

• **Medical Hx**:_____

_____

• **When/ where obtained**:   Date:_____ ;   □Breeder, □Shelter, Other:_____

Drug/ Suppl.	Amount	Dose (mg/kg)	Route	Frequency	Date Started

• **Vaccine status – Dog**: □Rab □Parv □Dist □Aden; □Para □Lep □Bord □Influ □Lyme
• **Vaccine status – Cat**: □Rab □Herp □Cali □Pan □FeLV[kittens]; □FIV □Chlam □Bord
• **Heartworm / Flea & Tick / Intestinal Parasites**:
  ◦ *Last Heartworm Test*: Date:_____, □IDK; Test Results: □Pos, □Neg, □IDK
  ◦ *Monthly heartworm preventative*:   □no □yes, Product:_____
  ◦ *Monthly flea & tick preventative*:   □no □yes, Product:_____
  ◦ *Monthly dewormer*:   □no □yes, Product:_____
• **Surgical Hx**:   □Spay/Neuter; Date:_____; Other:_____
• **Environment**: □Indoor, □Outdoor, Time spent outdoors/ Other:_____
• **Housemates**: Dogs:_____ Cats:_____ Other:_____
• **Diet**: □Wet, □Dry; Brand/ Amt.:_____

Appetite	□Normal, □↑, □↓
Weight	□Normal, □↑, □↓; Past Wt.:_____ kg; Date:_____ ; Δ:_____
Thirst	□Normal, □↑, □↓
Urination	□Normal, □↑, □↓, □Blood, □Strain
Defecation	□Normal, □↑, □↓, □Blood, □Strain, □Diarrhea, □Mucus
Discharge	□No, □Yes; Onset/ Describe:
Cough/ Sneeze	□No, □Yes; Onset/ Describe:
Vomit	□No, □Yes; Onset/ Describe:
Respiration	□Normal, □↑ Rate, □↑ Effort
Energy level	□Normal, □Lethargic, □Exercise intolerance

• **Travel Hx**: □None, Other:_____
• **Exposure to**: □Standing water, □Wildlife, □Board/daycare, □Dog park, □Groomer
• **Adverse reactions to food/ meds**: □None, Other:_____
• **Can give oral meds**: □no □yes; Helpful Tricks:_____

Physical Exam – General:

- **Body Weight**:_____kg   **Body Condition Score**:_____/9

- **Temperature**:_____°F [*Dog-RI*: 100.9–102.4; *Cat-RI*: 98.1–102.1]

- **Heart**:
  - *Rate*:_____beats/min [Dog-RI: 60–180; Cat-RI: 140–240 (in hospital)]
  - *Rhythm*: ☐Regular, ☐Irregular
  - *Sounds*: ☐None, ☐Split sound, ☐Gallop, ☐Murmur, ☐Muffled
    - *Grade*: ☐1–2[soft, only at PMI], ☐3–4[moderate, mild radiate], ☐5–6[strong radiate, thrill]
    - *Timing*: ☐Systolic, ☐Diastolic, ☐Continuous
    - *PMI*:

	PMI	Over	Anatomic Boundaries
☐	Lt. apex	Mitral valve	5th to 6th ICS at level of CCJ
☐	Lt. base	Ao + Pul outflow	2nd to 4th ICS above the CCJ
☐	Rt. midheart	Tricuspid valve	3rd to 5th ICS near the CCJ
☐	Rt. sternal border	Right ventricle	5th to 7th ICS immediately dorsal to the sternum
☐	Sternal (cat)	Sternum	In cats, PMI offers very little clinical significance.

  - • *Vertebral Heart Size*: Dog = 8.7–10.5; Cat = 6.9–8.1 (from cranial edge of T4)
  - • *Innocent Murmur*: Grade 1-2, systolic, left base location, disappear by ~4 months of age, absent clinical signs

- **Pulses**:
  - *Pulse rate*:_____pulses/min
  - *Character*: ☐Sync, ☐Async; ☐Normokinetic, ☐Hyper-, ☐Hypo-, ☐Variable

- **Lungs**:
  - *Respiratory rate*:_____breaths/min [*RI*: 16–30]
  - *Depth/Effort*: ☐Norm, ☐Pant, ☐Deep, ☐Shallow, ☐↑ Insp effort, ☐↑ Exp effort
  - *Sounds/Localization*:
    - ☐Norm BV, ☐Quiet BV, ☐Loud BV, ☐Crack, ☐Wheez, ☐Frict, ☐Muffled
    - ☐All fields, ☐Rt cran, ☐Rt mid, ☐Rt caud, ☐Lt cran, ☐Lt mid, ☐Lt caud
  - *Tracheal Auscultation/ Palpation*: ☐Normal, Other:_____

- **Pain Score**:_____ / 5   Localization:_____

- **Mentation**: ☐BAR   ☐Confused/   ☐Drowsy/   ☐Stuporous   ☐Coma
  ☐QAR   Disoriented   Obtunded   (unresponsive
  ☐Dull   unless aroused by
                                             noxious stimuli)

- **Skin Elasticity**: ☐Normal skin turgor, ☐↓ Skin turgor, ☐Skin tent, ☐Gelatinous

- **Mucus Membranes**:
  - *CRT*:_____ [*RI*: 1–2; <1 = compensated shock, sepsis, heat stroke; <2 = acute decompensated shock; >2 = late decompensated shock, decreased cardiac output, hypothermia]
  - *Color*:_____ [*RI*: pink; red = compensated shock, sepsis, heat stroke; pale/white = anemia, shock; blue = cyanosis; yellow = hepatic disease, extravascular hemolysis; brown = met-Hb]
  - *Texture*:_____ [*RI*: moist = hydrated; tacky-to-dry = 5–12% dehydrated]

Physical Exam – Systems Checklist:

- Head:_____ ☐NAF
  - Ears: ☐Debris (mild / mod / sev) (AS / AD / AU), _____ ☐NAF
  - Eyes:_____ ☐NAF
    - Retinal:_____ ☐NAF

	L →		R		L		R ←
☐	Normal Direct	☐	Normal Indirect	☐	Normal Indirect	☐	Normal Direct
☐	Abnormal Direct	☐	Abnormal Indirect	☐	Abnormal Indirect	☐	Abnormal Direct

  - Nose:_____ ☐NAF
  - Oral cavity: ☐Tarter/Gingivitis (mild / mod / sev), _____ ☐NAF
  - Mandibular lnn.: ☐Enlarged Lt., ☐Enlarged Rt., _____ ☐NAF

- Neck:_____ ☐NAF
  - Superficial cervical lnn.: ☐Enlarged Lt., ☐Enlarged Rt., _____ ☐NAF
  - Thyroid:_____ ☐NAF

- Thoracic limb:_____ ☐NAF
  - Foot pads:_____ ☐NAF
  - Knuckling:_____ ☐NAF
  - Axillary lnn. [normally absent]:_____ ☐NAF

- Thorax:_____ ☐NAF

- Abdomen:_____ ☐NAF
  - Mammary chain:_____ ☐NAF
  - Penis/ Testicles/ Vulva:_____ ☐NAF
  - Superficial inguinal lnn. [normally absent]:_____ ☐NAF

- Pelvic limb:_____ ☐NAF
  - Foot pads:_____ ☐NAF
  - Knuckling:_____ ☐NAF
  - Popliteal lnn.: ☐Enlarged Lt., ☐Enlarged Rt., _____ ☐NAF

- Skin:_____ ☐NAF
- Tail:_____ ☐NAF
- Rectal☞☉:_____ ☐NAF

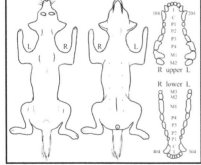
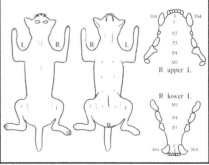

Problems List:

• **Problem #1**:

• **Problem #2**:

• **Problem #3**:

• **Problem #4**:

• **Problem #5**:

Diagnostic Plan	Treatment Plan

Case No._____

Patient	Age	Sex	Breed	Weight
	DOB:	Mn / Mi Fs / Fi	Color:	kg

Owner	Primary Veterinarian	Admit Date/ Time
Name: Phone:	Name: Phone:	Date: Time: AM / PM

• **Presenting Complaint**:_____
_____
_____

• **Medical Hx**:_____
_____
_____

• **When/ where obtained**:   Date:_____; ☐Breeder, ☐Shelter, Other:_____

Drug/ Suppl.	Amount	Dose (mg/kg)	Route	Frequency	Date Started

• **Vaccine status – Dog**: ☐Rab ☐Parv ☐Dist ☐Aden; ☐Para ☐Lep ☐Bord ☐Influ ☐Lyme
• **Vaccine status – Cat**: ☐Rab ☐Herp ☐Cali ☐Pan ☐FeLV[kittens]; ☐FIV ☐Chlam ☐Bord
• **Heartworm / Flea & Tick / Intestinal Parasites**:
  ◦ *Last Heartworm Test*: Date:_____, ☐IDK; Test Results: ☐Pos, ☐Neg, ☐IDK
  ◦ *Monthly heartworm preventative*: ☐no ☐yes, Product:_____
  ◦ *Monthly flea & tick preventative*: ☐no ☐yes, Product:_____
  ◦ *Monthly dewormer*:   ☐no ☐yes, Product:_____
• **Surgical Hx**: ☐Spay/Neuter; Date:_____; Other:_____
• **Environment**: ☐Indoor, ☐Outdoor, Time spent outdoors/ Other:_____
• **Housemates**: Dogs:_____ Cats:_____ Other:_____
• **Diet**: ☐Wet, ☐Dry; Brand/ Amt.:_____

Appetite	☐Normal, ☐↑, ☐↓
Weight	☐Normal, ☐↑, ☐↓; Past Wt.:_____ kg; Date:_____; Δ:_____
Thirst	☐Normal, ☐↑, ☐↓
Urination	☐Normal, ☐↑, ☐↓, ☐Blood, ☐Strain
Defecation	☐Normal, ☐↑, ☐↓, ☐Blood, ☐Strain, ☐Diarrhea, ☐Mucus
Discharge	☐No, ☐Yes; Onset/ Describe:
Cough/ Sneeze	☐No, ☐Yes; Onset/ Describe:
Vomit	☐No, ☐Yes; Onset/ Describe:
Respiration	☐Normal, ☐↑ Rate, ☐↑ Effort
Energy level	☐Normal, ☐Lethargic, ☐Exercise intolerance

• **Travel Hx**: ☐None, Other:_____
• **Exposure to**: ☐Standing water, ☐Wildlife, ☐Board/daycare, ☐Dog park, ☐Groomer
• **Adverse reactions to food/ meds**: ☐None, Other:_____
• **Can give oral meds**: ☐no ☐yes; Helpful Tricks:_____

Physical Exam – General:

- **Body Weight**:_____kg   **Body Condition Score**:_____/9

- **Temperature**:_____°F [*Dog-RI*: 100.9–102.4; *Cat-RI*: 98.1–102.1]

- **Heart**:
  - *Rate*:_____beats/min [Dog-RI: 60–180; Cat-RI: 140–240 (in hospital)]
  - *Rhythm*: □Regular, □Irregular
  - *Sounds*: □None, □Split sound, □Gallop, □Murmur, □Muffled
    - *Grade*: □1–2[soft, only at PMI], □3–4[moderate, mild radiate], □5–6[strong radiate, thrill]
    - *Timing*: □Systolic, □Diastolic, □Continuous
    - *PMI*:

	PMI	Over	Anatomic Boundaries
□	Lt. apex	Mitral valve	5th to 6th ICS at level of CCJ
□	Lt. base	Ao + Pul outflow	2nd to 4th ICS above the CCJ
□	Rt. midheart	Tricuspid valve	3rd to 5th ICS near the CCJ
□	Rt. sternal border	Right ventricle	5th to 7th ICS immediately dorsal to the sternum
□	Sternal (cat)	Sternum	In cats, PMI offers very little clinical significance.

   - •   *Vertebral Heart Size*: Dog = 8.7–10.5; Cat = 6.9–8.1 (from cranial edge of T4)
   - •   *Innocent Murmur*: Grade 1-2, systolic, left base location, disappear by ~4 months of age, absent clinical signs

- **Pulses**:
  - *Pulse rate*:_____pulses/min
  - *Character*: □Sync, □Async; □Normokinetic, □Hyper-, □Hypo-, □Variable

- **Lungs**:
  - *Respiratory rate*:_____breaths/min [*RI*: 16–30]
  - *Depth/Effort*: □Norm, □Pant, □Deep, □Shallow, □↑ Insp effort, □↑ Exp effort
  - *Sounds/Localization*:
    - □Norm BV, □Quiet BV, □Loud BV, □Crack, □Wheez, □Frict, □Muffled
    - □All fields, □Rt cran, □Rt mid, □Rt caud, □Lt cran, □Lt mid, □Lt caud
  - *Tracheal Auscultation/ Palpation*: □Normal, Other:_____

- **Pain Score**:_____ / 5   Localization:_____

- **Mentation**: □BAR   □Confused/   □Drowsy/   □Stuporous   □Coma
                □QAR   Disoriented   Obtunded   (unresponsive
                □Dull   unless aroused by
                                                       noxious stimuli)

- **Skin Elasticity**: □Normal skin turgor, □↓ Skin turgor, □Skin tent, □Gelatinous

- **Mucus Membranes**:
  - *CRT*:_____ [*RI*: 1–2; <1 = compensated shock, sepsis, heat stroke; <2 = acute decompensated shock; >2 = late decompensated shock, decreased cardiac output, hypothermia]
  - *Color*:_____ [*RI*: pink; red = compensated shock, sepsis, heat stroke; pale/white = anemia, shock; blue = cyanosis; yellow = hepatic disease, extravascular hemolysis; brown = met-Hb]
  - *Texture*:_____ [*RI*: moist = hydrated; tacky-to-dry = 5–12% dehydrated]

Physical Exam – Systems Checklist:

- Head:_____ ☐NAF
  - ∘ Ears: ☐Debris (mild / mod / sev) (AS / AD / AU),_____ ☐NAF
  - ∘ Eyes:_____ ☐NAF
    - ▪ Retinal:_____ ☐NAF

	→●Ⓛ		●Ⓡ		●Ⓛ		●Ⓡ←
☐	Normal Direct	☐	Normal Indirect	☐	Normal Indirect	☐	Normal Direct
☐	Abnormal Direct	☐	Abnormal Indirect	☐	Abnormal Indirect	☐	Abnormal Direct

  - ∘ Nose:_____ ☐NAF
  - ∘ Oral cavity: ☐Tarter/Gingivitis (mild / mod / sev),_____ ☐NAF
  - ∘ Mandibular lnn.: ☐Enlarged Lt., ☐Enlarged Rt.,_____ ☐NAF

- Neck:_____ ☐NAF
  - ∘ Superficial cervical lnn.: ☐Enlarged Lt., ☐Enlarged Rt.,_____ ☐NAF
  - ∘ Thyroid:_____ ☐NAF

- Thoracic limb:_____ ☐NAF
  - ∘ Foot pads:_____ ☐NAF
  - ∘ Knuckling:_____ ☐NAF
  - ∘ Axillary lnn. [normally absent]:_____ ☐NAF

- Thorax:_____ ☐NAF

- Abdomen:_____ ☐NAF
  - ∘ Mammary chain:_____ ☐NAF
  - ∘ Penis/ Testicles/ Vulva:_____ ☐NAF
  - ∘ Superficial inguinal lnn. [normally absent]:_____ ☐NAF

- Pelvic limb:_____ ☐NAF
  - ∘ Foot pads:_____ ☐NAF
  - ∘ Knuckling:_____ ☐NAF
  - ∘ Popliteal lnn.: ☐Enlarged Lt., ☐Enlarged Rt.,_____ ☐NAF

- Skin:_____ ☐NAF
- Tail:_____ ☐NAF
- Rectal☞☉:_____ ☐NAF

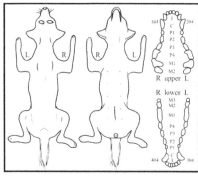 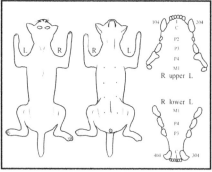

Problems List:

• Problem #1:

• Problem #2:

• Problem #3:

• Problem #4:

• Problem #5:

Diagnostic Plan	Treatment Plan

Case No._____

Patient	Age	Sex	Breed	Weight
	DOB:	Mn / Mi Fs / Fi	Color:	kg

Owner		Primary Veterinarian	Admit Date/ Time
Name: Phone:		Name: Phone:	Date: Time: AM / PM

• **Presenting Complaint**:_____
_____
_____

• **Medical Hx**:_____
_____
_____

• **When/ where obtained**:   Date:_____; □Breeder, □Shelter, Other:_____

Drug/ Suppl.	Amount	Dose (mg/kg)	Route	Frequency	Date Started

• **Vaccine status – Dog**: □Rab □Parv □Dist □Aden; □Para □Lep □Bord □Influ □Lyme
• **Vaccine status – Cat**: □Rab □Herp □Cali □Pan □FeLV[kittens]; □FIV □Chlam □Bord
• **Heartworm / Flea & Tick / Intestinal Parasites**:
   ◦ *Last Heartworm Test*: Date:_____, □IDK; Test Results: □Pos, □Neg, □IDK
   ◦ *Monthly heartworm preventative*:   □no □yes, Product:_____
   ◦ *Monthly flea & tick preventative*:   □no □yes, Product:_____
   ◦ *Monthly dewormer*:   □no □yes, Product:_____
• **Surgical Hx**:   □Spay/Neuter; Date:_____; Other:_____
• **Environment**: □Indoor, □Outdoor, Time spent outdoors/ Other:_____
• **Housemates**: Dogs:_____ Cats:_____ Other:_____
• **Diet**: □Wet, □Dry; Brand/ Amt.:_____

Appetite	□Normal, □↑, □↓
Weight	□Normal, □↑, □↓; Past Wt.:_____ kg; Date:_____; Δ:_____
Thirst	□Normal, □↑, □↓
Urination	□Normal, □↑, □↓, □Blood, □Strain
Defecation	□Normal, □↑, □↓, □Blood, □Strain, □Diarrhea, □Mucus
Discharge	□No, □Yes; Onset/ Describe:
Cough/ Sneeze	□No, □Yes; Onset/ Describe:
Vomit	□No, □Yes; Onset/ Describe:
Respiration	□Normal, □↑ Rate, □↑ Effort
Energy level	□Normal, □Lethargic, □Exercise intolerance

• **Travel Hx**: □None, Other:_____
• **Exposure to**: □Standing water, □Wildlife, □Board/daycare, □Dog park, □Groomer
• **Adverse reactions to food/ meds**: □None, Other:_____
• **Can give oral meds**: □no □yes; Helpful Tricks:_____

Physical Exam – General:

• **Body Weight**:_____kg   **Body Condition Score**:_____/9

• **Temperature**:_____°F [*Dog-RI*: 100.9–102.4; *Cat-RI*: 98.1–102.1]

• **Heart**:
- *Rate*:_____beats/min [Dog-RI: 60–180; Cat-RI: 140–240 (in hospital)]
- *Rhythm*:   □Regular, □Irregular
- *Sounds*:   □None, □Split sound, □Gallop, □Murmur, □Muffled
   - *Grade*:   □1–2[soft, only at PMI],   □3–4[moderate, mild radiate],   □5–6[strong radiate, thrill]
   - *Timing*: □Systolic, □Diastolic, □Continuous
   - *PMI*:

	PMI	Over	Anatomic Boundaries
□	Lt. apex	Mitral valve	5th to 6th ICS at level of CCJ
□	Lt. base	Ao + Pul outflow	2nd to 4th ICS above the CCJ
□	Rt. midheart	Tricuspid valve	3rd to 5th ICS near the CCJ
□	Rt. sternal border	Right ventricle	5th to 7th ICS immediately dorsal to the sternum
□	Sternal (cat)	Sternum	In cats, PMI offers very little clinical significance.

   - • *Vertebral Heart Size*: Dog = 8.7–10.5; Cat = 6.9–8.1 (from cranial edge of T4)
   - • *Innocent Murmur*: Grade 1-2, systolic, left base location, disappear by ~4 months of age, absent clinical signs

• **Pulses**:
- *Pulse rate*:_____pulses/min
- *Character*:   □Sync, □Async;   □Normokinetic, □Hyper-, □Hypo-, □Variable

• **Lungs**:
- *Respiratory rate*:_____breaths/min [*RI*: 16–30]
- *Depth/Effort*: □Norm, □Pant, □Deep, □Shallow, □↑ Insp effort, □↑ Exp effort
- *Sounds/Localization*:
   - □Norm BV, □Quiet BV, □Loud BV, □Crack, □Wheez, □Frict, □Muffled
   - □All fields, □Rt cran, □Rt mid, □Rt caud, □Lt cran, □Lt mid, □Lt caud
- *Tracheal Auscultation/ Palpation*: □Normal, Other:_____

• **Pain Score**:_____ / 5   Localization:_____

• **Mentation**: □BAR   □Confused/   □Drowsy/   □Stuporous   □Coma
                 □QAR   Disoriented   Obtunded   (unresponsive
                 □Dull   unless aroused by
                                                             noxious stimuli)

• **Skin Elasticity**: □Normal skin turgor, □↓ Skin turgor, □Skin tent, □Gelatinous

• **Mucus Membranes**:
- *CRT*:_____ [*RI*: 1–2; <1 = compensated shock, sepsis, heat stroke; <2 = acute decompensated shock; >2 = late decompensated shock, decreased cardiac output, hypothermia]
- *Color*:_____ [*RI*: pink; red = compensated shock, sepsis, heat stroke; pale/white = anemia, shock; blue = cyanosis; yellow = hepatic disease, extravascular hemolysis; brown = met-Hb]
- *Texture*:_____ [*RI*: moist = hydrated; tacky-to-dry = 5–12% dehydrated]

Physical Exam – Systems Checklist:

- Head:_____ ☐NAF
  - Ears: ☐Debris (mild / mod / sev) (AS / AD / AU), _____ ☐NAF
  - Eyes:_____ ☐NAF
    - Retinal:_____ ☐NAF

	→ ⓛ		ⓡ		ⓛ		ⓡ ←
☐	Normal Direct	☐	Normal Indirect	☐	Normal Indirect	☐	Normal Direct
☐	Abnormal Direct	☐	Abnormal Indirect	☐	Abnormal Indirect	☐	Abnormal Direct

  - Nose:_____ ☐NAF
  - Oral cavity: ☐Tarter/Gingivitis (mild / mod / sev), _____ ☐NAF
  - Mandibular lnn.: ☐Enlarged Lt., ☐Enlarged Rt., _____ ☐NAF

- Neck:_____ ☐NAF
  - Superficial cervical lnn.: ☐Enlarged Lt., ☐Enlarged Rt., _____ ☐NAF
  - Thyroid:_____ ☐NAF

- Thoracic limb:_____ ☐NAF
  - Foot pads:_____ ☐NAF
  - Knuckling:_____ ☐NAF
  - Axillary lnn. [normally absent]:_____ ☐NAF

- Thorax:_____ ☐NAF

- Abdomen:_____ ☐NAF
  - Mammary chain:_____ ☐NAF
  - Penis/ Testicles/ Vulva:_____ ☐NAF
  - Superficial inguinal lnn. [normally absent]:_____ ☐NAF

- Pelvic limb:_____ ☐NAF
  - Foot pads:_____ ☐NAF
  - Knuckling:_____ ☐NAF
  - Popliteal lnn.: ☐Enlarged Lt., ☐Enlarged Rt., _____ ☐NAF

- Skin:_____ ☐NAF
- Tail:_____ ☐NAF
- Rectal☞☉:_____ ☐NAF

• **Problem #1**:

• **Problem #2**:

• **Problem #3**:

• **Problem #4**:

• **Problem #5**:

Diagnostic Plan	Treatment Plan

Case No._____

Patient	Age	Sex	Breed	Weight
	DOB:	Mn / Mi Fs / Fi	Color:	kg

Owner	Primary Veterinarian	Admit Date/ Time
Name: Phone:	Name: Phone:	Date: Time: AM / PM

• **Presenting Complaint**:_____

_____

• **Medical Hx**:_____

_____

• **When/ where obtained**:   Date:_____ ;   ☐Breeder, ☐Shelter, Other:_____

Drug/ Suppl.	Amount	Dose (mg/kg)	Route	Frequency	Date Started

• **Vaccine status – Dog**: ☐Rab ☐Parv ☐Dist ☐Aden; ☐Para ☐Lep ☐Bord ☐Influ ☐Lyme
• **Vaccine status – Cat**: ☐Rab ☐Herp ☐Cali ☐Pan ☐FeLV[kittens]; ☐FIV ☐Chlam ☐Bord
• **Heartworm / Flea & Tick / Intestinal Parasites**:
  ◦ *Last Heartworm Test*: Date:_____, ☐IDK; Test Results: ☐Pos, ☐Neg, ☐IDK
  ◦ *Monthly heartworm preventative*: ☐no ☐yes, Product:_____
  ◦ *Monthly flea & tick preventative*: ☐no ☐yes, Product:_____
  ◦ *Monthly dewormer*:   ☐no ☐yes, Product:_____
• **Surgical Hx**: ☐Spay/Neuter; Date:_____ ; Other:_____
• **Environment**: ☐Indoor, ☐Outdoor, Time spent outdoors/ Other:_____
• **Housemates**: Dogs:_____ Cats:_____ Other:_____
• **Diet**: ☐Wet, ☐Dry; Brand/ Amt.:_____

Appetite	☐Normal, ☐↑, ☐↓
Weight	☐Normal, ☐↑, ☐↓; Past Wt.:_____ kg; Date:_____ ; Δ:_____
Thirst	☐Normal, ☐↑, ☐↓
Urination	☐Normal, ☐↑, ☐↓, ☐Blood, ☐Strain
Defecation	☐Normal, ☐↑, ☐↓, ☐Blood, ☐Strain, ☐Diarrhea, ☐Mucus
Discharge	☐No, ☐Yes; Onset/ Describe:
Cough/ Sneeze	☐No, ☐Yes; Onset/ Describe:
Vomit	☐No, ☐Yes; Onset/ Describe:
Respiration	☐Normal, ☐↑ Rate, ☐↑ Effort
Energy level	☐Normal, ☐Lethargic, ☐Exercise intolerance

• **Travel Hx**: ☐None, Other:_____
• **Exposure to**: ☐Standing water, ☐Wildlife, ☐Board/daycare, ☐Dog park, ☐Groomer
• **Adverse reactions to food/ meds**: ☐None, Other:_____
• **Can give oral meds**: ☐no ☐yes; Helpful Tricks:_____

Physical Exam – General:

- **Body Weight**:_____kg **Body Condition Score**:_____/9

- **Temperature**:_____°F [*Dog-RI*: 100.9–102.4; *Cat-RI*: 98.1–102.1]

- **Heart**:
  - *Rate*:_____beats/min [Dog-RI: 60–180; Cat-RI: 140–240 (in hospital)]
  - *Rhythm*: □Regular, □Irregular
  - *Sounds*: □None, □Split sound, □Gallop, □Murmur, □Muffled
    - *Grade*: □1–2[soft, only at PMI], □3–4[moderate, mild radiate], □5–6[strong radiate, thrill]
    - *Timing*: □Systolic, □Diastolic, □Continuous
    - *PMI*:

	PMI	Over	Anatomic Boundaries
□	Lt. apex	Mitral valve	5th to 6th ICS at level of CCJ
□	Lt. base	Ao + Pul outflow	2nd to 4th ICS above the CCJ
□	Rt. midheart	Tricuspid valve	3rd to 5th ICS near the CCJ
□	Rt. sternal border	Right ventricle	5th to 7th ICS immediately dorsal to the sternum
□	Sternal (cat)	Sternum	In cats, PMI offers very little clinical significance.

- *Vertebral Heart Size*: Dog = 8.7–10.5; Cat = 6.9–8.1 (from cranial edge of T4)
- *Innocent Murmur*: Grade 1-2, systolic, left base location, disappear by ~4 months of age, absent clinical signs

- **Pulses**:
  - *Pulse rate*:_____pulses/min
  - *Character*: □Sync, □Async; □Normokinetic, □Hyper-, □Hypo-, □Variable

- **Lungs**:
  - *Respiratory rate*:_____breaths/min [*RI*: 16–30]
  - *Depth/Effort*: □Norm, □Pant, □Deep, □Shallow, □↑ Insp effort, □↑ Exp effort
  - *Sounds/Localization*:
    - □Norm BV, □Quiet BV, □Loud BV, □Crack, □Wheez, □Frict, □Muffled
    - □All fields, □Rt cran, □Rt mid, □Rt caud, □Lt cran, □Lt mid, □Lt caud
  - *Tracheal Auscultation/ Palpation*: □Normal, Other:_____

- **Pain Score**:_____ / 5   Localization:_____

- **Mentation**: □BAR   □Confused/   □Drowsy/   □Stuporous   □Coma
  □QAR   Disoriented   Obtunded   (unresponsive
  □Dull   unless aroused by
                                                              noxious stimuli)

- **Skin Elasticity**: □Normal skin turgor, □↓ Skin turgor, □Skin tent, □Gelatinous

- **Mucus Membranes**:
  - *CRT*:_____ [*RI*: 1–2; <1 = compensated shock, sepsis, heat stroke; <2 = acute decompensated shock; >2 = late decompensated shock, decreased cardiac output, hypothermia]
  - *Color*:_____ [*RI*: pink; red = compensated shock, sepsis, heat stroke; pale/white = anemia, shock; blue = cyanosis; yellow = hepatic disease, extravascular hemolysis; brown = met-Hb]
  - *Texture*:_____ [*RI*: moist = hydrated; tacky-to-dry = 5–12% dehydrated]

<u>Physical Exam – Systems Checklist</u>:

• Head:_____ ☐NAF
   ◦ Ears: ☐Debris (mild / mod / sev) (AS / AD / AU),_____ ☐NAF
   ◦ Eyes:_____ ☐NAF
     ▪ Retinal:_____ ☐NAF

→ ⓛ		ⓡ		ⓛ		ⓡ ←	
☐	Normal Direct	☐	Normal Indirect	☐	Normal Indirect	☐	Normal Direct
☐	Abnormal Direct	☐	Abnormal Indirect	☐	Abnormal Indirect	☐	Abnormal Direct

   ◦ Nose:_____ ☐NAF
   ◦ Oral cavity: ☐Tarter/Gingivitis (mild / mod / sev),_____ ☐NAF
   ◦ Mandibular lnn.: ☐Enlarged Lt., ☐Enlarged Rt.,_____ ☐NAF

• Neck:_____ ☐NAF
   ◦ Superficial cervical lnn.: ☐Enlarged Lt., ☐Enlarged Rt.,_____ ☐NAF
   ◦ Thyroid:_____ ☐NAF

• Thoracic limb:_____ ☐NAF
   ◦ Foot pads:_____ ☐NAF
   ◦ Knuckling:_____ ☐NAF
   ◦ Axillary lnn. [normally absent]:_____ ☐NAF

• Thorax:_____ ☐NAF

• Abdomen:_____ ☐NAF
   ◦ Mammary chain:_____ ☐NAF
   ◦ Penis/ Testicles/ Vulva:_____ ☐NAF
   ◦ Superficial inguinal lnn. [normally absent]:_____ ☐NAF

• Pelvic limb:_____ ☐NAF
   ◦ Foot pads:_____ ☐NAF
   ◦ Knuckling:_____ ☐NAF
   ◦ Popliteal lnn.: ☐Enlarged Lt., ☐Enlarged Rt.,_____ ☐NAF

• Skin:_____ ☐NAF
• Tail:_____ ☐NAF
• Rectal☞☉:_____ ☐NAF

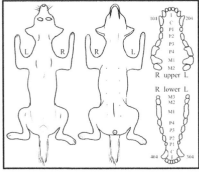
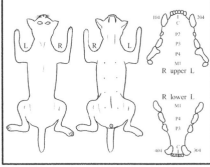

<u>**Problems List**</u>:

• Problem #1:

• Problem #2:

• Problem #3:

• Problem #4:

• Problem #5:

Diagnostic Plan	Treatment Plan

Case No._____

Patient	Age	Sex	Breed	Weight
	DOB:	Mn / Mi Fs / Fi	Color:	kg

Owner	Primary Veterinarian	Admit Date/ Time
Name: Phone:	Name: Phone:	Date: Time: AM / PM

• **Presenting Complaint**:_____
_____
_____

• **Medical Hx**:_____
_____
_____

• **When/ where obtained**: Date:_____; □Breeder, □Shelter, Other:_____

Drug/ Suppl.	Amount	Dose (mg/kg)	Route	Frequency	Date Started

• **Vaccine status – Dog**: □Rab □Parv □Dist □Aden; □Para □Lep □Bord □Influ □Lyme
• **Vaccine status – Cat**: □Rab □Herp □Cali □Pan □FeLV[kittens]; □FIV □Chlam □Bord
• **Heartworm / Flea & Tick / Intestinal Parasites**:
  ◦ *Last Heartworm Test*: Date:_____, □IDK; Test Results: □Pos, □Neg, □IDK
  ◦ *Monthly heartworm preventative*:   □no □yes, Product:_____
  ◦ *Monthly flea & tick preventative*:   □no □yes, Product:_____
  ◦ *Monthly dewormer*:   □no □yes, Product:_____
• **Surgical Hx**: □Spay/Neuter; Date:_____; Other:_____
• **Environment**: □Indoor, □Outdoor, Time spent outdoors/ Other:_____
• **Housemates**: Dogs:_____ Cats:_____ Other:_____
• **Diet**: □Wet, □Dry; Brand/ Amt.:_____

Appetite	□Normal, □↑, □↓
Weight	□Normal, □↑, □↓; Past Wt.:_____ kg; Date:_____; Δ:_____
Thirst	□Normal, □↑, □↓
Urination	□Normal, □↑, □↓, □Blood, □Strain
Defecation	□Normal, □↑, □↓, □Blood, □Strain, □Diarrhea, □Mucus
Discharge	□No, □Yes; Onset/ Describe:
Cough/ Sneeze	□No, □Yes; Onset/ Describe:
Vomit	□No, □Yes; Onset/ Describe:
Respiration	□Normal, □↑ Rate, □↑ Effort
Energy level	□Normal, □Lethargic, □Exercise intolerance

• **Travel Hx**: □None, Other:_____
• **Exposure to**: □Standing water, □Wildlife, □Board/daycare, □Dog park, □Groomer
• **Adverse reactions to food/ meds**: □None, Other:_____
• **Can give oral meds**: □no □yes; Helpful Tricks:_____

Physical Exam – General:

- **Body Weight:**_____kg   **Body Condition Score:**_____/9

- **Temperature:**_____°F [*Dog-RI*: 100.9–102.4; *Cat-RI*: 98.1–102.1]

- **Heart:**
  - *Rate*:_____beats/min [Dog-RI: 60–180; Cat-RI: 140–240 (in hospital)]
  - *Rhythm*: ☐Regular, ☐Irregular
  - *Sounds*: ☐None, ☐Split sound, ☐Gallop, ☐Murmur, ☐Muffled
    - *Grade*: ☐1–2[soft, only at PMI], ☐3–4[moderate, mild radiate], ☐5–6[strong radiate, thrill]
    - *Timing*: ☐Systolic, ☐Diastolic, ☐Continuous
    - *PMI*:

	PMI	Over	Anatomic Boundaries
☐	Lt. apex	Mitral valve	5th to 6th ICS at level of CCJ
☐	Lt. base	Ao + Pul outflow	2nd to 4th ICS above the CCJ
☐	Rt. midheart	Tricuspid valve	3rd to 5th ICS near the CCJ
☐	Rt. sternal border	Right ventricle	5th to 7th ICS immediately dorsal to the sternum
☐	Sternal (cat)	Sternum	In cats, PMI offers very little clinical significance.

   - *Vertebral Heart Size*: Dog = 8.7–10.5; Cat = 6.9–8.1 (from cranial edge of T4)
   - *Innocent Murmur*: Grade 1-2, systolic, left base location, disappear by ~4 months of age, absent clinical signs

- **Pulses:**
  - *Pulse rate*:_____pulses/min
  - *Character*: ☐Sync, ☐Async; ☐Normokinetic, ☐Hyper-, ☐Hypo-, ☐Variable

- **Lungs:**
  - *Respiratory rate*:_____breaths/min [*RI*: 16–30]
  - *Depth/Effort*: ☐Norm, ☐Pant, ☐Deep, ☐Shallow, ☐↑ Insp effort, ☐↑ Exp effort
  - *Sounds/Localization*:
    - ☐Norm BV, ☐Quiet BV, ☐Loud BV, ☐Crack, ☐Wheez, ☐Frict, ☐Muffled
    - ☐All fields, ☐Rt cran, ☐Rt mid, ☐Rt caud, ☐Lt cran, ☐Lt mid, ☐Lt caud
  - *Tracheal Auscultation/ Palpation*: ☐Normal, Other:_____

- **Pain Score:**_____ / 5   Localization:_____

- **Mentation:** ☐BAR   ☐Confused/   ☐Drowsy/   ☐Stuporous   ☐Coma
            ☐QAR   Disoriented   Obtunded   (unresponsive
            ☐Dull   unless aroused by
                                              noxious stimuli)

- **Skin Elasticity:** ☐Normal skin turgor, ☐↓ Skin turgor, ☐Skin tent, ☐Gelatinous

- **Mucus Membranes:**
  - *CRT*:_____ [*RI*: 1–2; <1 = compensated shock, sepsis, heat stroke; <2 = acute decompensated shock; >2 = late decompensated shock, decreased cardiac output, hypothermia]
  - *Color*:_____ [*RI*: pink; red = compensated shock, sepsis, heat stroke; pale/white = anemia, shock; blue = cyanosis; yellow = hepatic disease, extravascular hemolysis; brown = met-Hb]
  - *Texture*:_____ [*RI*: moist = hydrated; tacky-to-dry = 5–12% dehydrated]

Physical Exam – Systems Checklist:

- Head:_____ ☐NAF
  - ◦ Ears: ☐Debris (mild / mod / sev) (AS / AD / AU), _____ ☐NAF
  - ◦ Eyes:_____ ☐NAF
    - ▪ Retinal:_____ ☐NAF

→ ⓛ		ⓡ		ⓛ		ⓡ ←	
☐	Normal Direct	☐	Normal Indirect	☐	Normal Indirect	☐	Normal Direct
☐	Abnormal Direct	☐	Abnormal Indirect	☐	Abnormal Indirect	☐	Abnormal Direct

  - ◦ Nose:_____ ☐NAF
  - ◦ Oral cavity: ☐Tarter/Gingivitis (mild / mod / sev), _____ ☐NAF
  - ◦ Mandibular lnn.: ☐Enlarged Lt., ☐Enlarged Rt., _____ ☐NAF

- Neck:_____ ☐NAF
  - ◦ Superficial cervical lnn.: ☐Enlarged Lt., ☐Enlarged Rt., _____ ☐NAF
  - ◦ Thyroid:_____ ☐NAF

- Thoracic limb:_____ ☐NAF
  - ◦ Foot pads:_____ ☐NAF
  - ◦ Knuckling:_____ ☐NAF
  - ◦ Axillary lnn. [normally absent]:_____ ☐NAF

- Thorax:_____ ☐NAF

- Abdomen:_____ ☐NAF
  - ◦ Mammary chain:_____ ☐NAF
  - ◦ Penis/ Testicles/ Vulva:_____ ☐NAF
  - ◦ Superficial inguinal lnn. [normally absent]:_____ ☐NAF

- Pelvic limb:_____ ☐NAF
  - ◦ Foot pads:_____ ☐NAF
  - ◦ Knuckling:_____ ☐NAF
  - ◦ Popliteal lnn.: ☐Enlarged Lt., ☐Enlarged Rt., _____ ☐NAF

- Skin:_____ ☐NAF
- Tail:_____ ☐NAF
- Rectal☞☉:_____ ☐NAF

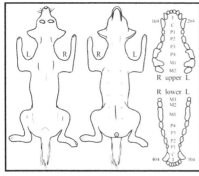

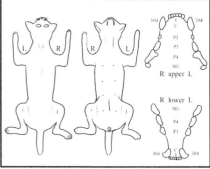

Problems List:

• **Problem #1**:

• **Problem #2**:

• **Problem #3**:

• **Problem #4**:

• **Problem #5**:

Diagnostic Plan	Treatment Plan

Case No._____

Patient	Age	Sex	Breed	Weight
	DOB:	Mn / Mi Fs / Fi	Color:	kg

Owner	Primary Veterinarian	Admit Date/ Time
Name: Phone:	Name: Phone:	Date: Time: AM / PM

• **Presenting Complaint**:_____

_____

• **Medical Hx**:_____

_____

• **When/ where obtained**:   Date:_____;   ☐Breeder, ☐Shelter, Other:_____

Drug/ Suppl.	Amount	Dose (mg/kg)	Route	Frequency	Date Started

• **Vaccine status – Dog**: ☐Rab ☐Parv ☐Dist ☐Aden; ☐Para ☐Lep ☐Bord ☐Influ ☐Lyme
• **Vaccine status – Cat**: ☐Rab ☐Herp ☐Cali ☐Pan ☐FeLV[kittens]; ☐FIV ☐Chlam ☐Bord
• **Heartworm / Flea & Tick / Intestinal Parasites**:
  ◦ *Last Heartworm Test*: Date:_____, ☐IDK; Test Results: ☐Pos, ☐Neg, ☐IDK
  ◦ *Monthly heartworm preventative*:   ☐no ☐yes, Product:_____
  ◦ *Monthly flea & tick preventative*:   ☐no ☐yes, Product:_____
  ◦ *Monthly dewormer*:   ☐no ☐yes, Product:_____
• **Surgical Hx**:   ☐Spay/Neuter; Date:_____;   Other:_____
• **Environment**: ☐Indoor, ☐Outdoor, Time spent outdoors/ Other:_____
• **Housemates**: Dogs:_____ Cats:_____ Other:_____
• **Diet**: ☐Wet, ☐Dry; Brand/ Amt.:_____

Appetite	☐Normal, ☐↑, ☐↓
Weight	☐Normal, ☐↑, ☐↓; Past Wt.:_____ kg; Date:_____; Δ:_____
Thirst	☐Normal, ☐↑, ☐↓
Urination	☐Normal, ☐↑, ☐↓, ☐Blood, ☐Strain
Defecation	☐Normal, ☐↑, ☐↓, ☐Blood, ☐Strain, ☐Diarrhea, ☐Mucus
Discharge	☐No, ☐Yes; Onset/ Describe:
Cough/ Sneeze	☐No, ☐Yes; Onset/ Describe:
Vomit	☐No, ☐Yes; Onset/ Describe:
Respiration	☐Normal, ☐↑ Rate, ☐↑ Effort
Energy level	☐Normal, ☐Lethargic, ☐Exercise intolerance

• **Travel Hx**: ☐None, Other:_____
• **Exposure to**: ☐Standing water, ☐Wildlife, ☐Board/daycare, ☐Dog park, ☐Groomer
• **Adverse reactions to food/ meds**: ☐None, Other:_____
• **Can give oral meds**: ☐no ☐yes; Helpful Tricks:_____

Physical Exam – General:

- **Body Weight**:_____kg **Body Condition Score**:_____/9

- **Temperature**:_____°F [*Dog-RI*: 100.9–102.4; *Cat-RI*: 98.1–102.1]

- **Heart**:
  - *Rate*:_____beats/min [Dog-RI: 60–180; Cat-RI: 140–240 (in hospital)]
  - *Rhythm*: ☐Regular, ☐Irregular
  - *Sounds*: ☐None, ☐Split sound, ☐Gallop, ☐Murmur, ☐Muffled
    - *Grade*: ☐1–2[soft, only at PMI], ☐3–4[moderate, mild radiate], ☐5–6[strong radiate, thrill]
    - *Timing*: ☐Systolic, ☐Diastolic, ☐Continuous
    - *PMI*:

	PMI	Over	Anatomic Boundaries
☐	Lt. apex	Mitral valve	5th to 6th ICS at level of CCJ
☐	Lt. base	Ao + Pul outflow	2nd to 4th ICS above the CCJ
☐	Rt. midheart	Tricuspid valve	3rd to 5th ICS near the CCJ
☐	Rt. sternal border	Right ventricle	5th to 7th ICS immediately dorsal to the sternum
☐	Sternal (cat)	Sternum	In cats, PMI offers very little clinical significance.

  - • *Vertebral Heart Size*: Dog = 8.7–10.5; Cat = 6.9–8.1 (from cranial edge of T4)
  - • *Innocent Murmur*: Grade 1-2, systolic, left base location, disappear by ~4 months of age, absent clinical signs

- **Pulses**:
  - *Pulse rate*:_____pulses/min
  - *Character*: ☐Sync, ☐Async; ☐Normokinetic, ☐Hyper-, ☐Hypo-, ☐Variable

- **Lungs**:
  - *Respiratory rate*:_____breaths/min [*RI*: 16–30]
  - *Depth/Effort*: ☐Norm, ☐Pant, ☐Deep, ☐Shallow, ☐↑ Insp effort, ☐↑ Exp effort
  - *Sounds/Localization*:
    - ☐Norm BV, ☐Quiet BV, ☐Loud BV, ☐Crack, ☐Wheez, ☐Frict, ☐Muffled
    - ☐All fields, ☐Rt cran, ☐Rt mid, ☐Rt caud, ☐Lt cran, ☐Lt mid, ☐Lt caud
  - *Tracheal Auscultation/ Palpation*: ☐Normal, Other:_____

- **Pain Score**:_____ / 5   Localization:_____

- **Mentation**: ☐BAR ☐Confused/ ☐Drowsy/ ☐Stuporous ☐Coma
                 ☐QAR   Disoriented Obtunded (unresponsive
                 ☐Dull   unless aroused by
                                               noxious stimuli)

- **Skin Elasticity**: ☐Normal skin turgor, ☐↓ Skin turgor, ☐Skin tent, ☐Gelatinous

- **Mucus Membranes**:
  - *CRT*:_____ [*RI*: 1–2; <1 = compensated shock, sepsis, heat stroke; <2 = acute decompensated shock; >2 = late decompensated shock, decreased cardiac output, hypothermia]
  - *Color*:_____ [*RI*: pink; red = compensated shock, sepsis, heat stroke; pale/white = anemia, shock; blue = cyanosis; yellow = hepatic disease, extravascular hemolysis; brown = met-Hb]
  - *Texture*:_____ [*RI*: moist = hydrated; tacky-to-dry = 5–12% dehydrated]

Physical Exam – Systems Checklist:

- Head:_____ ☐NAF
  - ◦ Ears: ☐Debris (mild / mod / sev) (AS / AD / AU),_____ ☐NAF
  - ◦ Eyes:_____ ☐NAF
    - ▪ Retinal:_____ ☐NAF

→ ⓛ		ⓡ		ⓛ		ⓡ ←	
☐	Normal Direct	☐	Normal Indirect	☐	Normal Indirect	☐	Normal Direct
☐	Abnormal Direct	☐	Abnormal Indirect	☐	Abnormal Indirect	☐	Abnormal Direct

  - ◦ Nose:_____ ☐NAF
  - ◦ Oral cavity: ☐Tarter/Gingivitis (mild / mod / sev),_____ ☐NAF
  - ◦ Mandibular lnn.: ☐Enlarged Lt., ☐Enlarged Rt.,_____ ☐NAF

- Neck:_____ ☐NAF
  - ◦ Superficial cervical lnn.: ☐Enlarged Lt., ☐Enlarged Rt.,_____ ☐NAF
  - ◦ Thyroid:_____ ☐NAF

- Thoracic limb:_____ ☐NAF
  - ◦ Foot pads:_____ ☐NAF
  - ◦ Knuckling:_____ ☐NAF
  - ◦ Axillary lnn. [normally absent]:_____ ☐NAF

- Thorax:_____ ☐NAF

- Abdomen:_____ ☐NAF
  - ◦ Mammary chain:_____ ☐NAF
  - ◦ Penis/ Testicles/ Vulva:_____ ☐NAF
  - ◦ Superficial inguinal lnn. [normally absent]:_____ ☐NAF

- Pelvic limb:_____ ☐NAF
  - ◦ Foot pads:_____ ☐NAF
  - ◦ Knuckling:_____ ☐NAF
  - ◦ Popliteal lnn.: ☐Enlarged Lt., ☐Enlarged Rt.,_____ ☐NAF

- Skin:_____ ☐NAF
- Tail:_____ ☐NAF
- Rectal☞☉:_____ ☐NAF

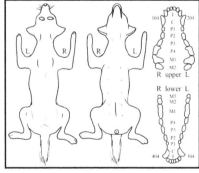
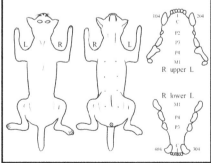

Problems List:

• **Problem #1**:

• **Problem #2**:

• **Problem #3**:

• **Problem #4**:

• **Problem #5**:

Diagnostic Plan	Treatment Plan

Case No._____

Patient	Age	Sex	Breed	Weight
	DOB:	Mn / Mi Fs / Fi	Color:	kg

Owner	Primary Veterinarian	Admit Date/ Time
Name: Phone:	Name: Phone:	Date: Time: AM / PM

• **Presenting Complaint**:_____

• **Medical Hx**:_____

• **When/ where obtained**: Date:_____ ; □Breeder, □Shelter, Other:_____

Drug/ Suppl.	Amount	Dose (mg/kg)	Route	Frequency	Date Started

• **Vaccine status – Dog**: □Rab □Parv □Dist □Aden; □Para □Lep □Bord □Influ □Lyme
• **Vaccine status – Cat**: □Rab □Herp □Cali □Pan □FeLV[kittens]; □FIV □Chlam □Bord
• **Heartworm / Flea & Tick / Intestinal Parasites**:
   ◦ *Last Heartworm Test*: Date:_____, □IDK; Test Results: □Pos, □Neg, □IDK
   ◦ *Monthly heartworm preventative*: □no □yes, Product:_____
   ◦ *Monthly flea & tick preventative*: □no □yes, Product:_____
   ◦ *Monthly dewormer*: □no □yes, Product:_____
• **Surgical Hx**: □Spay/Neuter; Date:_____; Other:_____
• **Environment**: □Indoor, □Outdoor, Time spent outdoors/ Other:_____
• **Housemates**: Dogs:_____ Cats:_____ Other:_____
• **Diet**: □Wet, □Dry; Brand/ Amt.:_____

Appetite	□Normal, □↑, □↓
Weight	□Normal, □↑, □↓; Past Wt.:_____ kg; Date:_____ ; Δ:_____
Thirst	□Normal, □↑, □↓
Urination	□Normal, □↑, □↓, □Blood, □Strain
Defecation	□Normal, □↑, □↓, □Blood, □Strain, □Diarrhea, □Mucus
Discharge	□No, □Yes; Onset/ Describe:
Cough/ Sneeze	□No, □Yes; Onset/ Describe:
Vomit	□No, □Yes; Onset/ Describe:
Respiration	□Normal, □↑ Rate, □↑ Effort
Energy level	□Normal, □Lethargic, □Exercise intolerance

• **Travel Hx**: □None, Other:_____
• **Exposure to**: □Standing water, □Wildlife, □Board/daycare, □Dog park, □Groomer
• **Adverse reactions to food/ meds**: □None, Other:_____
• **Can give oral meds**: □no □yes; Helpful Tricks:_____

Physical Exam – General:

- **Body Weight**:_____kg   **Body Condition Score**:_____/9

- **Temperature**:_____°F [*Dog-RI*: 100.9–102.4; *Cat-RI*: 98.1–102.1]

- **Heart**:
  - *Rate*:_____beats/min [Dog-RI: 60–180; Cat-RI: 140–240 (in hospital)]
  - *Rhythm*:   ☐Regular, ☐Irregular
  - *Sounds*:   ☐None, ☐Split sound, ☐Gallop, ☐Murmur, ☐Muffled
    - *Grade*:   ☐1–2[soft, only at PMI],   ☐3–4[moderate, mild radiate],   ☐5–6[strong radiate, thrill]
    - *Timing*: ☐Systolic, ☐Diastolic, ☐Continuous
    - *PMI*:

	PMI	Over	Anatomic Boundaries
☐	Lt. apex	Mitral valve	5th to 6th ICS at level of CCJ
☐	Lt. base	Ao + Pul outflow	2nd to 4th ICS above the CCJ
☐	Rt. midheart	Tricuspid valve	3rd to 5th ICS near the CCJ
☐	Rt. sternal border	Right ventricle	5th to 7th ICS immediately dorsal to the sternum
☐	Sternal (cat)	Sternum	In cats, PMI offers very little clinical significance.

- *Vertebral Heart Size*: Dog = 8.7–10.5; Cat = 6.9–8.1 (from cranial edge of T4)
- *Innocent Murmur*: Grade 1-2, systolic, left base location, disappear by ~4 months of age, absent clinical signs

- **Pulses**:
  - *Pulse rate*:_____pulses/min
  - *Character*:   ☐Sync, ☐Async;   ☐Normokinetic, ☐Hyper-, ☐Hypo-, ☐Variable

- **Lungs**:
  - *Respiratory rate*:_____breaths/min [*RI*: 16–30]
  - *Depth/Effort*: ☐Norm, ☐Pant, ☐Deep, ☐Shallow, ☐↑ Insp effort, ☐↑ Exp effort
  - *Sounds/Localization*:
    - ☐Norm BV, ☐Quiet BV, ☐Loud BV, ☐Crack, ☐Wheez, ☐Frict, ☐Muffled
    - ☐All fields, ☐Rt cran, ☐Rt mid, ☐Rt caud, ☐Lt cran, ☐Lt mid, ☐Lt caud
  - *Tracheal Auscultation/ Palpation*: ☐Normal, Other:_____

- **Pain Score**:_____ / 5   Localization:_____

- **Mentation**: ☐BAR   ☐Confused/   ☐Drowsy/   ☐Stuporous   ☐Coma
                 ☐QAR   Disoriented   Obtunded   (unresponsive
                 ☐Dull   unless aroused by
                                                            noxious stimuli)

- **Skin Elasticity**: ☐Normal skin turgor, ☐↓ Skin turgor, ☐Skin tent, ☐Gelatinous

- **Mucus Membranes**:
  - *CRT*:_____ [*RI*: 1–2; <1 = compensated shock, sepsis, heat stroke; <2 = acute decompensated shock; >2 = late decompensated shock, decreased cardiac output, hypothermia]
  - *Color*:_____ [*RI*: pink; red = compensated shock, sepsis, heat stroke; pale/white = anemia, shock; blue = cyanosis; yellow = hepatic disease, extravascular hemolysis; brown = met-Hb]
  - *Texture*:_____ [*RI*: moist = hydrated; tacky-to-dry = 5–12% dehydrated]

Physical Exam – Systems Checklist:

- Head:_____ ☐NAF
  - Ears: ☐Debris (mild / mod / sev) (AS / AD / AU),_____ ☐NAF
  - Eyes:_____ ☐NAF
    - Retinal:_____ ☐NAF

→ Ⓛ	Ⓡ	Ⓛ	Ⓡ ←
☐ Normal Direct	☐ Normal Indirect	☐ Normal Indirect	☐ Normal Direct
☐ Abnormal Direct	☐ Abnormal Indirect	☐ Abnormal Indirect	☐ Abnormal Direct

  - Nose:_____ ☐NAF
  - Oral cavity: ☐Tarter/Gingivitis (mild / mod / sev),_____ ☐NAF
  - Mandibular lnn.: ☐Enlarged Lt., ☐Enlarged Rt.,_____ ☐NAF

- Neck:_____ ☐NAF
  - Superficial cervical lnn.: ☐Enlarged Lt., ☐Enlarged Rt.,_____ ☐NAF
  - Thyroid:_____ ☐NAF

- Thoracic limb:_____ ☐NAF
  - Foot pads:_____ ☐NAF
  - Knuckling:_____ ☐NAF
  - Axillary lnn. [normally absent]:_____ ☐NAF

- Thorax:_____ ☐NAF

- Abdomen:_____ ☐NAF
  - Mammary chain:_____ ☐NAF
  - Penis/ Testicles/ Vulva:_____ ☐NAF
  - Superficial inguinal lnn. [normally absent]:_____ ☐NAF

- Pelvic limb:_____ ☐NAF
  - Foot pads:_____ ☐NAF
  - Knuckling:_____ ☐NAF
  - Popliteal lnn.: ☐Enlarged Lt., ☐Enlarged Rt.,_____ ☐NAF

- Skin:_____ ☐NAF
- Tail:_____ ☐NAF
- Rectal☞☉:_____ ☐NAF

142

<u>**Problems List**</u>:

• **Problem #1**:

• **Problem #2**:

• **Problem #3**:

• **Problem #4**:

• **Problem #5**:

Diagnostic Plan	Treatment Plan

Case No._____

Patient	Age	Sex	Breed	Weight
	DOB:	Mn / Mi Fs / Fi	Color:	kg

Owner		Primary Veterinarian	Admit Date/ Time
Name: Phone:		Name: Phone:	Date: Time: AM / PM

• **Presenting Complaint**:_____

_____

• **Medical Hx**:_____

_____

• **When/ where obtained**: Date:_____; ☐Breeder, ☐Shelter, Other:_____

Drug/ Suppl.	Amount	Dose (mg/kg)	Route	Frequency	Date Started

• **Vaccine status – Dog**: ☐Rab ☐Parv ☐Dist ☐Aden; ☐Para ☐Lep ☐Bord ☐Influ ☐Lyme
• **Vaccine status – Cat**: ☐Rab ☐Herp ☐Cali ☐Pan ☐FeLV[kittens]; ☐FIV ☐Chlam ☐Bord
• **Heartworm / Flea & Tick / Intestinal Parasites**:
  ◦ *Last Heartworm Test*: Date:_____, ☐IDK; Test Results: ☐Pos, ☐Neg, ☐IDK
  ◦ *Monthly heartworm preventative*:   ☐no ☐yes, Product:_____
  ◦ *Monthly flea & tick preventative*:   ☐no ☐yes, Product:_____
  ◦ *Monthly dewormer*:   ☐no ☐yes, Product:_____
• **Surgical Hx**: ☐Spay/Neuter; Date:_____; Other:_____
• **Environment**: ☐Indoor, ☐Outdoor, Time spent outdoors/ Other:_____
• **Housemates**: Dogs:_____ Cats:_____ Other:_____
• **Diet**: ☐Wet, ☐Dry; Brand/ Amt.:_____

Appetite	☐Normal, ☐↑, ☐↓
Weight	☐Normal, ☐↑, ☐↓; Past Wt.:_____ kg; Date:_____; Δ:_____
Thirst	☐Normal, ☐↑, ☐↓
Urination	☐Normal, ☐↑, ☐↓, ☐Blood, ☐Strain
Defecation	☐Normal, ☐↑, ☐↓, ☐Blood, ☐Strain, ☐Diarrhea, ☐Mucus
Discharge	☐No, ☐Yes; Onset/ Describe:
Cough/ Sneeze	☐No, ☐Yes; Onset/ Describe:
Vomit	☐No, ☐Yes; Onset/ Describe:
Respiration	☐Normal, ☐↑ Rate, ☐↑ Effort
Energy level	☐Normal, ☐Lethargic, ☐Exercise intolerance

• **Travel Hx**: ☐None, Other:_____
• **Exposure to**: ☐Standing water, ☐Wildlife, ☐Board/daycare, ☐Dog park, ☐Groomer
• **Adverse reactions to food/ meds**: ☐None, Other:_____
• **Can give oral meds**: ☐no ☐yes; Helpful Tricks:_____

144

Physical Exam – General:

- **Body Weight:** _____ kg   **Body Condition Score:** _____ /9

- **Temperature:** _____ °F [*Dog-RI*: 100.9–102.4; *Cat-RI*: 98.1–102.1]

- **Heart:**
  - *Rate:* _____ beats/min [Dog-RI: 60–180; Cat-RI: 140–240 (in hospital)]
  - *Rhythm:* ☐Regular, ☐Irregular
  - *Sounds:* ☐None, ☐Split sound, ☐Gallop, ☐Murmur, ☐Muffled
    - *Grade:* ☐1–2[soft, only at PMI], ☐3–4[moderate, mild radiate], ☐5–6[strong radiate, thrill]
    - *Timing:* ☐Systolic, ☐Diastolic, ☐Continuous
    - *PMI:*

	PMI	Over	Anatomic Boundaries
☐	Lt. apex	Mitral valve	5th to 6th ICS at level of CCJ
☐	Lt. base	Ao + Pul outflow	2nd to 4th ICS above the CCJ
☐	Rt. midheart	Tricuspid valve	3rd to 5th ICS near the CCJ
☐	Rt. sternal border	Right ventricle	5th to 7th ICS immediately dorsal to the sternum
☐	Sternal (cat)	Sternum	In cats, PMI offers very little clinical significance.

  - *Vertebral Heart Size:* Dog = 8.7–10.5; Cat = 6.9–8.1 (from cranial edge of T4)
  - *Innocent Murmur:* Grade 1-2, systolic, left base location, disappear by ~4 months of age, absent clinical signs

- **Pulses:**
  - *Pulse rate:* _____ pulses/min
  - *Character:* ☐Sync, ☐Async; ☐Normokinetic, ☐Hyper-, ☐Hypo-, ☐Variable

- **Lungs:**
  - *Respiratory rate:* _____ breaths/min [*RI*: 16–30]
  - *Depth/Effort:* ☐Norm, ☐Pant, ☐Deep, ☐Shallow, ☐↑ Insp effort, ☐↑ Exp effort
  - *Sounds/Localization:*
    - ☐Norm BV, ☐Quiet BV, ☐Loud BV, ☐Crack, ☐Wheez, ☐Frict, ☐Muffled
    - ☐All fields, ☐Rt cran, ☐Rt mid, ☐Rt caud, ☐Lt cran, ☐Lt mid, ☐Lt caud
  - *Tracheal Auscultation/ Palpation:* ☐Normal, Other: _____

- **Pain Score:** _____ / 5   Localization: _____

- **Mentation:** ☐BAR   ☐Confused/   ☐Drowsy/   ☐Stuporous   ☐Coma
                 ☐QAR   Disoriented   Obtunded   (unresponsive
                 ☐Dull   unless aroused by
                                                           noxious stimuli)

- **Skin Elasticity:** ☐Normal skin turgor, ☐↓ Skin turgor, ☐Skin tent, ☐Gelatinous

- **Mucus Membranes:**
  - *CRT:* _____ [*RI*: 1–2; <1 = compensated shock, sepsis, heat stroke; <2 = acute decompensated shock; >2 = late decompensated shock, decreased cardiac output, hypothermia]
  - *Color:* _____ [*RI*: pink; red = compensated shock, sepsis, heat stroke; pale/white = anemia, shock; blue = cyanosis; yellow = hepatic disease, extravascular hemolysis; brown = met-Hb]
  - *Texture:* _____ [*RI*: moist = hydrated; tacky-to-dry = 5–12% dehydrated]

Physical Exam – Systems Checklist:

- Head:_____ ☐NAF
  - Ears: ☐Debris (mild / mod / sev) (AS / AD / AU),_____ ☐NAF
  - Eyes:_____ ☐NAF
    - Retinal:_____ ☐NAF

☐	Normal Direct	☐	Normal Indirect	☐	Normal Indirect	☐	Normal Direct
☐	Abnormal Direct	☐	Abnormal Indirect	☐	Abnormal Indirect	☐	Abnormal Direct

  - Nose:_____ ☐NAF
  - Oral cavity: ☐Tarter/Gingivitis (mild / mod / sev),_____ ☐NAF
  - Mandibular lnn.: ☐Enlarged Lt., ☐Enlarged Rt.,_____ ☐NAF

- Neck:_____ ☐NAF
  - Superficial cervical lnn.: ☐Enlarged Lt., ☐Enlarged Rt.,_____ ☐NAF
  - Thyroid:_____ ☐NAF

- Thoracic limb:_____ ☐NAF
  - Foot pads:_____ ☐NAF
  - Knuckling:_____ ☐NAF
  - Axillary lnn. [normally absent]:_____ ☐NAF

- Thorax:_____ ☐NAF

- Abdomen:_____ ☐NAF
  - Mammary chain:_____ ☐NAF
  - Penis/ Testicles/ Vulva:_____ ☐NAF
  - Superficial inguinal lnn. [normally absent]:_____ ☐NAF

- Pelvic limb:_____ ☐NAF
  - Foot pads:_____ ☐NAF
  - Knuckling:_____ ☐NAF
  - Popliteal lnn.: ☐Enlarged Lt., ☐Enlarged Rt.,_____ ☐NAF

- Skin:_____ ☐NAF
- Tail:_____ ☐NAF
- Rectal☞☉:_____ ☐NAF

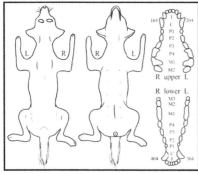
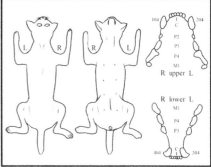

Problems List:

• **Problem #1**:

• **Problem #2**:

• **Problem #3**:

• **Problem #4**:

• **Problem #5**:

Diagnostic Plan	Treatment Plan

Case No._____

Patient	Age	Sex	Breed	Weight
	DOB:	Mn / Mi Fs / Fi	Color:	kg

Owner	Primary Veterinarian	Admit Date/ Time
Name: Phone:	Name: Phone:	Date: Time: AM / PM

• **Presenting Complaint**:_____

_____

• **Medical Hx**:_____

_____

• **When/ where obtained**:   Date:_____; ☐Breeder, ☐Shelter, Other:_____

Drug/ Suppl.	Amount	Dose (mg/kg)	Route	Frequency	Date Started

• **Vaccine status – Dog**: ☐Rab ☐Parv ☐Dist ☐Aden; ☐Para ☐Lep ☐Bord ☐Influ ☐Lyme
• **Vaccine status – Cat**: ☐Rab ☐Herp ☐Cali ☐Pan ☐FeLV[kittens]; ☐FIV ☐Chlam ☐Bord
• **Heartworm / Flea & Tick / Intestinal Parasites**:
  ◦ *Last Heartworm Test*: Date:_____, ☐IDK; Test Results: ☐Pos, ☐Neg, ☐IDK
  ◦ *Monthly heartworm preventative*: ☐no ☐yes, Product:_____
  ◦ *Monthly flea & tick preventative*: ☐no ☐yes, Product:_____
  ◦ *Monthly dewormer*: ☐no ☐yes, Product:_____
• **Surgical Hx**:   ☐Spay/Neuter; Date:_____; Other:_____
• **Environment**: ☐Indoor, ☐Outdoor, Time spent outdoors/ Other:_____
• **Housemates**: Dogs:_____ Cats:_____ Other:_____
• **Diet**: ☐Wet, ☐Dry; Brand/ Amt.:_____

Appetite	☐Normal, ☐↑, ☐↓
Weight	☐Normal, ☐↑, ☐↓; Past Wt.:_____ kg; Date:_____; Δ:_____
Thirst	☐Normal, ☐↑, ☐↓
Urination	☐Normal, ☐↑, ☐↓, ☐Blood, ☐Strain
Defecation	☐Normal, ☐↑, ☐↓, ☐Blood, ☐Strain, ☐Diarrhea, ☐Mucus
Discharge	☐No, ☐Yes; Onset/ Describe:
Cough/ Sneeze	☐No, ☐Yes; Onset/ Describe:
Vomit	☐No, ☐Yes; Onset/ Describe:
Respiration	☐Normal, ☐↑ Rate, ☐↑ Effort
Energy level	☐Normal, ☐Lethargic, ☐Exercise intolerance

• **Travel Hx**: ☐None, Other:_____
• **Exposure to**: ☐Standing water, ☐Wildlife, ☐Board/daycare, ☐Dog park, ☐Groomer
• **Adverse reactions to food/ meds**: ☐None, Other:_____
• **Can give oral meds**: ☐no ☐yes; Helpful Tricks:_____

Physical Exam – General:

- **Body Weight**:_____kg   **Body Condition Score**:_____/9

- **Temperature**:_____°F [*Dog-RI*: 100.9–102.4; *Cat-RI*: 98.1–102.1]

- **Heart**:
  - *Rate*:_____beats/min [Dog-RI: 60–180; Cat-RI: 140–240 (in hospital)]
  - *Rhythm*:   □Regular, □Irregular
  - *Sounds*:   □None, □Split sound, □Gallop, □Murmur, □Muffled
    - *Grade*:   □1–2[soft, only at PMI], □3–4[moderate, mild radiate], □5–6[strong radiate, thrill]
    - *Timing*: □Systolic, □Diastolic, □Continuous
    - *PMI*:

	PMI	Over	Anatomic Boundaries
□	Lt. apex	Mitral valve	5th to 6th ICS at level of CCJ
□	Lt. base	Ao + Pul outflow	2nd to 4th ICS above the CCJ
□	Rt. midheart	Tricuspid valve	3rd to 5th ICS near the CCJ
□	Rt. sternal border	Right ventricle	5th to 7th ICS immediately dorsal to the sternum
□	Sternal (cat)	Sternum	In cats, PMI offers very little clinical significance.

  - • *Vertebral Heart Size*: Dog = 8.7–10.5; Cat = 6.9–8.1 (from cranial edge of T4)
  - • *Innocent Murmur*: Grade 1-2, systolic, left base location, disappear by ~4 months of age, absent clinical signs

- **Pulses**:
  - *Pulse rate*:_____pulses/min
  - *Character*:   □Sync, □Async;   □Normokinetic, □Hyper-, □Hypo-, □Variable

- **Lungs**:
  - *Respiratory rate*:_____breaths/min [*RI*: 16–30]
  - *Depth/Effort*: □Norm, □Pant, □Deep, □Shallow, □↑ Insp effort, □↑ Exp effort
  - *Sounds/Localization*:
    - □Norm BV, □Quiet BV, □Loud BV, □Crack, □Wheez, □Frict, □Muffled
    - □All fields, □Rt cran, □Rt mid, □Rt caud, □Lt cran, □Lt mid, □Lt caud
  - *Tracheal Auscultation/ Palpation*: □Normal, Other:_____

- **Pain Score**:_____ / 5   Localization:_____

- **Mentation**: □BAR   □Confused/   □Drowsy/   □Stuporous   □Coma
                 □QAR   Disoriented   Obtunded   (unresponsive
                 □Dull   unless aroused by
                                                              noxious stimuli)

- **Skin Elasticity**: □Normal skin turgor, □↓ Skin turgor, □Skin tent, □Gelatinous

- **Mucus Membranes**:
  - *CRT*:_____ [*RI*: 1–2; <1 = compensated shock, sepsis, heat stroke; <2 = acute decompensated shock; >2 = late decompensated shock, decreased cardiac output, hypothermia]
  - *Color*:_____ [*RI*: pink; red = compensated shock, sepsis, heat stroke; pale/white = anemia, shock; blue = cyanosis; yellow = hepatic disease, extravascular hemolysis; brown = met-Hb]
  - *Texture*:_____ [*RI*: moist = hydrated; tacky-to-dry = 5–12% dehydrated]

Physical Exam – Systems Checklist:

- Head:_____ ☐NAF
  - Ears: ☐Debris (mild / mod / sev) (AS / AD / AU),_____ ☐NAF
  - Eyes:_____ ☐NAF
    - Retinal:_____ ☐NAF

☐	Normal Direct	☐	Normal Indirect	☐	Normal Indirect	☐	Normal Direct
☐	Abnormal Direct	☐	Abnormal Indirect	☐	Abnormal Indirect	☐	Abnormal Direct

  - Nose:_____ ☐NAF
  - Oral cavity: ☐Tarter/Gingivitis (mild / mod / sev),_____ ☐NAF
  - Mandibular lnn.: ☐Enlarged Lt., ☐Enlarged Rt.,_____ ☐NAF

- Neck:_____ ☐NAF
  - Superficial cervical lnn.: ☐Enlarged Lt., ☐Enlarged Rt.,_____ ☐NAF
  - Thyroid:_____ ☐NAF

- Thoracic limb:_____ ☐NAF
  - Foot pads:_____ ☐NAF
  - Knuckling:_____ ☐NAF
  - Axillary lnn. [normally absent]:_____ ☐NAF

- Thorax:_____ ☐NAF

- Abdomen:_____ ☐NAF
  - Mammary chain:_____ ☐NAF
  - Penis/ Testicles/ Vulva:_____ ☐NAF
  - Superficial inguinal lnn. [normally absent]:_____ ☐NAF

- Pelvic limb:_____ ☐NAF
  - Foot pads:_____ ☐NAF
  - Knuckling:_____ ☐NAF
  - Popliteal lnn.: ☐Enlarged Lt., ☐Enlarged Rt.,_____ ☐NAF

- Skin:_____ ☐NAF
- Tail:_____ ☐NAF
- Rectal☞☉:_____ ☐NAF

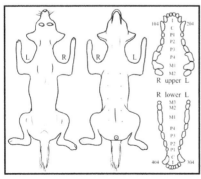

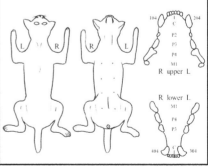

Problems List:

• **Problem #1**:

• **Problem #2**:

• **Problem #3**:

• **Problem #4**:

• **Problem #5**:

Diagnostic Plan	Treatment Plan

Patient	Age	Sex	Breed	Weight
	DOB:	Mn / Mi Fs / Fi	Color:	kg

Owner	Primary Veterinarian	Admit Date/ Time
Name: Phone:	Name: Phone:	Date: Time: AM / PM

• **Presenting Complaint**:_____
_____
_____

• **Medical Hx**:_____
_____
_____

• **When/ where obtained**:   Date:_____ ;   □Breeder, □Shelter, Other:_____

Drug/ Suppl.	Amount	Dose (mg/kg)	Route	Frequency	Date Started

• **Vaccine status – Dog**: □Rab □Parv □Dist □Aden; □Para □Lep □Bord □Influ □Lyme
• **Vaccine status – Cat**: □Rab □Herp □Cali □Pan □FeLV[kittens]; □FIV □Chlam □Bord
• **Heartworm / Flea & Tick / Intestinal Parasites**:
    ◦ *Last Heartworm Test*: Date:_____, □IDK; Test Results: □Pos, □Neg, □IDK
    ◦ *Monthly heartworm preventative*: □no □yes, Product:_____
    ◦ *Monthly flea & tick preventative*: □no □yes, Product:_____
    ◦ *Monthly dewormer*:   □no □yes, Product:_____
• **Surgical Hx**:   □Spay/Neuter; Date:_____ ;   Other:_____
• **Environment**: □Indoor, □Outdoor, Time spent outdoors/ Other:_____
• **Housemates**: Dogs:_____ Cats:_____ Other:_____
• **Diet**: □Wet, □Dry; Brand/ Amt.:_____

Appetite	□Normal, □↑, □↓
Weight	□Normal, □↑, □↓; Past Wt.:_____ kg; Date:_____; Δ:_____
Thirst	□Normal, □↑, □↓
Urination	□Normal, □↑, □↓, □Blood, □Strain
Defecation	□Normal, □↑, □↓, □Blood, □Strain, □Diarrhea, □Mucus
Discharge	□No, □Yes; Onset/ Describe:
Cough/ Sneeze	□No, □Yes; Onset/ Describe:
Vomit	□No, □Yes; Onset/ Describe:
Respiration	□Normal, □↑ Rate, □↑ Effort
Energy level	□Normal, □Lethargic, □Exercise intolerance

• **Travel Hx**: □None, Other:_____
• **Exposure to**: □Standing water, □Wildlife, □Board/daycare, □Dog park, □Groomer
• **Adverse reactions to food/ meds**: □None, Other:_____
• **Can give oral meds**: □no □yes; Helpful Tricks:_____

Physical Exam – General:

- **Body Weight**:_____kg   **Body Condition Score**:_____/9

- **Temperature**:_____°F [*Dog-RI*: 100.9–102.4; *Cat-RI*: 98.1–102.1]

- **Heart**:
  - *Rate*:_____beats/min [Dog-RI: 60–180; Cat-RI: 140–240 (in hospital)]
  - *Rhythm*:   ☐Regular, ☐Irregular
  - *Sounds*:   ☐None, ☐Split sound, ☐Gallop, ☐Murmur, ☐Muffled
    - *Grade*:   ☐1–2[soft, only at PMI],   ☐3–4[moderate, mild radiate],   ☐5–6[strong radiate, thrill]
    - *Timing*: ☐Systolic, ☐Diastolic, ☐Continuous
    - *PMI*:

	PMI	Over	Anatomic Boundaries
☐	Lt. apex	Mitral valve	5th to 6th ICS at level of CCJ
☐	Lt. base	Ao + Pul outflow	2nd to 4th ICS above the CCJ
☐	Rt. midheart	Tricuspid valve	3rd to 5th ICS near the CCJ
☐	Rt. sternal border	Right ventricle	5th to 7th ICS immediately dorsal to the sternum
☐	Sternal (cat)	Sternum	In cats, PMI offers very little clinical significance.

-     *Vertebral Heart Size*: Dog = 8.7–10.5; Cat = 6.9–8.1 (from cranial edge of T4)
-     *Innocent Murmur*: Grade 1-2, systolic, left base location, disappear by ~4 months of age, absent clinical signs

- **Pulses**:
  - *Pulse rate*:_____pulses/min
  - *Character*:   ☐Sync, ☐Async;   ☐Normokinetic, ☐Hyper-, ☐Hypo-, ☐Variable

- **Lungs**:
  - *Respiratory rate*:_____breaths/min [*RI*: 16–30]
  - *Depth/Effort*: ☐Norm, ☐Pant, ☐Deep, ☐Shallow, ☐↑ Insp effort, ☐↑ Exp effort
  - *Sounds/Localization*:
    - ☐Norm BV, ☐Quiet BV, ☐Loud BV, ☐Crack, ☐Wheez, ☐Frict, ☐Muffled
    - ☐All fields, ☐Rt cran, ☐Rt mid, ☐Rt caud, ☐Lt cran, ☐Lt mid, ☐Lt caud
  - *Tracheal Auscultation/ Palpation*: ☐Normal, Other:_____

- **Pain Score**:_____ / 5   Localization:_____

- **Mentation**: ☐BAR   ☐Confused/   ☐Drowsy/   ☐Stuporous   ☐Coma
                ☐QAR   Disoriented   Obtunded   (unresponsive
                ☐Dull   unless aroused by
                                                 noxious stimuli)

- **Skin Elasticity**: ☐Normal skin turgor, ☐↓ Skin turgor, ☐Skin tent, ☐Gelatinous

- **Mucus Membranes**:
  - *CRT*:_____ [*RI*: 1–2; <1 = compensated shock, sepsis, heat stroke; <2 = acute decompensated shock; >2 = late decompensated shock, decreased cardiac output, hypothermia]
  - *Color*:_____ [*RI*: pink; red = compensated shock, sepsis, heat stroke; pale/white = anemia, shock; blue = cyanosis; yellow = hepatic disease, extravascular hemolysis; brown = met-Hb]
  - *Texture*:_____ [*RI*: moist = hydrated; tacky-to-dry = 5–12% dehydrated]

Physical Exam – Systems Checklist:

- Head:_____ ☐NAF
  - Ears: ☐Debris (mild / mod / sev) (AS / AD / AU),_____ ☐NAF
  - Eyes:_____ ☐NAF
    - Retinal:_____ ☐NAF

☐	Normal Direct	☐	Normal Indirect	☐	Normal Indirect	☐	Normal Direct
☐	Abnormal Direct	☐	Abnormal Indirect	☐	Abnormal Indirect	☐	Abnormal Direct

  - Nose:_____ ☐NAF
  - Oral cavity: ☐Tarter/Gingivitis (mild / mod / sev),_____ ☐NAF
  - Mandibular lnn.: ☐Enlarged Lt., ☐Enlarged Rt.,_____ ☐NAF

- Neck:_____ ☐NAF
  - Superficial cervical lnn.: ☐Enlarged Lt., ☐Enlarged Rt.,_____ ☐NAF
  - Thyroid:_____ ☐NAF

- Thoracic limb:_____ ☐NAF
  - Foot pads:_____ ☐NAF
  - Knuckling:_____ ☐NAF
  - Axillary lnn. [normally absent]:_____ ☐NAF

- Thorax:_____ ☐NAF

- Abdomen:_____ ☐NAF
  - Mammary chain:_____ ☐NAF
  - Penis/ Testicles/ Vulva:_____ ☐NAF
  - Superficial inguinal lnn. [normally absent]:_____ ☐NAF

- Pelvic limb:_____ ☐NAF
  - Foot pads:_____ ☐NAF
  - Knuckling:_____ ☐NAF
  - Popliteal lnn.: ☐Enlarged Lt., ☐Enlarged Rt.,_____ ☐NAF

- Skin:_____ ☐NAF
- Tail:_____ ☐NAF
- Rectal☞⊙:_____ ☐NAF

Problems List:

• **Problem #1**:

• **Problem #2**:

• **Problem #3**:

• **Problem #4**:

• **Problem #5**:

Diagnostic Plan	Treatment Plan

Case No._____

Patient	Age	Sex	Breed	Weight
	DOB:	Mn / Mi Fs / Fi	Color:	kg

Owner	Primary Veterinarian	Admit Date/ Time
Name: Phone:	Name: Phone:	Date: Time: AM / PM

• **Presenting Complaint**:_____
_____
_____

• **Medical Hx**:_____
_____
_____

• **When/ where obtained**: Date:_____; □Breeder, □Shelter, Other:_____

Drug/ Suppl.	Amount	Dose (mg/kg)	Route	Frequency	Date Started

• **Vaccine status – Dog**: □Rab □Parv □Dist □Aden; □Para □Lep □Bord □Influ □Lyme
• **Vaccine status – Cat**: □Rab □Herp □Cali □Pan □FeLV[kittens]; □FIV □Chlam □Bord
• **Heartworm / Flea & Tick / Intestinal Parasites**:
  ◦ *Last Heartworm Test*: Date:_____, □IDK; Test Results: □Pos, □Neg, □IDK
  ◦ *Monthly heartworm preventative*:   □no □yes, Product:_____
  ◦ *Monthly flea & tick preventative*:   □no □yes, Product:_____
  ◦ *Monthly dewormer*:   □no □yes, Product:_____
• **Surgical Hx**: □Spay/Neuter; Date:_____; Other:_____
• **Environment**: □Indoor, □Outdoor, Time spent outdoors/ Other:_____
• **Housemates**: Dogs:_____ Cats:_____ Other:_____
• **Diet**: □Wet, □Dry; Brand/ Amt.:_____

Appetite	□Normal, □↑, □↓
Weight	□Normal, □↑, □↓; Past Wt.:_____ kg; Date:_____; Δ:_____
Thirst	□Normal, □↑, □↓
Urination	□Normal, □↑, □↓, □Blood, □Strain
Defecation	□Normal, □↑, □↓, □Blood, □Strain, □Diarrhea, □Mucus
Discharge	□No, □Yes; Onset/ Describe:
Cough/ Sneeze	□No, □Yes; Onset/ Describe:
Vomit	□No, □Yes; Onset/ Describe:
Respiration	□Normal, □↑ Rate, □↑ Effort
Energy level	□Normal, □Lethargic, □Exercise intolerance

• **Travel Hx**: □None, Other:_____
• **Exposure to**: □Standing water, □Wildlife, □Board/daycare, □Dog park, □Groomer
• **Adverse reactions to food/ meds**: □None, Other:_____
• **Can give oral meds**: □no □yes; Helpful Tricks:_____

Physical Exam – General:

- **Body Weight**:_____kg **Body Condition Score**:_____/9

- **Temperature**:_____°F [*Dog-RI*: 100.9–102.4; *Cat-RI*: 98.1–102.1]

- **Heart**:
  - *Rate*:_____beats/min [Dog-RI: 60–180; Cat-RI: 140–240 (in hospital)]
  - *Rhythm*: ☐Regular, ☐Irregular
  - *Sounds*: ☐None, ☐Split sound, ☐Gallop, ☐Murmur, ☐Muffled
    - *Grade*: ☐1–2[soft, only at PMI], ☐3–4[moderate, mild radiate], ☐5–6[strong radiate, thrill]
    - *Timing*: ☐Systolic, ☐Diastolic, ☐Continuous
    - *PMI*:

	PMI	Over	Anatomic Boundaries
☐	Lt. apex	Mitral valve	5th to 6th ICS at level of CCJ
☐	Lt. base	Ao + Pul outflow	2nd to 4th ICS above the CCJ
☐	Rt. midheart	Tricuspid valve	3rd to 5th ICS near the CCJ
☐	Rt. sternal border	Right ventricle	5th to 7th ICS immediately dorsal to the sternum
☐	Sternal (cat)	Sternum	In cats, PMI offers very little clinical significance.

- *Vertebral Heart Size*: Dog = 8.7–10.5; Cat = 6.9–8.1 (from cranial edge of T4)
- *Innocent Murmur*: Grade 1-2, systolic, left base location, disappear by ~4 months of age, absent clinical signs

- **Pulses**:
  - *Pulse rate*:_____pulses/min
  - *Character*: ☐Sync, ☐Async; ☐Normokinetic, ☐Hyper-, ☐Hypo-, ☐Variable

- **Lungs**:
  - *Respiratory rate*:_____breaths/min [*RI*: 16–30]
  - *Depth/Effort*: ☐Norm, ☐Pant, ☐Deep, ☐Shallow, ☐↑ Insp effort, ☐↑ Exp effort
  - *Sounds/Localization*:
    - ☐Norm BV, ☐Quiet BV, ☐Loud BV, ☐Crack, ☐Wheez, ☐Frict, ☐Muffled
    - ☐All fields, ☐Rt cran, ☐Rt mid, ☐Rt caud, ☐Lt cran, ☐Lt mid, ☐Lt caud
  - *Tracheal Auscultation/ Palpation*: ☐Normal, Other:_____

- **Pain Score**:_____ / 5   Localization:_____

- **Mentation**: ☐BAR ☐Confused/ ☐Drowsy/ ☐Stuporous ☐Coma
  ☐QAR Disoriented Obtunded (unresponsive
  ☐Dull unless aroused by
  noxious stimuli)

- **Skin Elasticity**: ☐Normal skin turgor, ☐↓ Skin turgor, ☐Skin tent, ☐Gelatinous

- **Mucus Membranes**:
  - *CRT*:_____ [*RI*: 1–2; <1 = compensated shock, sepsis, heat stroke; <2 = acute decompensated shock; >2 = late decompensated shock, decreased cardiac output, hypothermia]
  - *Color*:_____ [*RI*: pink; red = compensated shock, sepsis, heat stroke; pale/white = anemia, shock; blue = cyanosis; yellow = hepatic disease, extravascular hemolysis; brown = met-Hb]
  - *Texture*:_____ [*RI*: moist = hydrated; tacky-to-dry = 5–12% dehydrated]

Physical Exam – Systems Checklist:

- Head:_____ ☐NAF
  - Ears: ☐Debris (mild / mod / sev) (AS / AD / AU),_____ ☐NAF
  - Eyes:_____ ☐NAF
    - Retinal:_____ ☐NAF

	→ ⊙ L		⊙ R		⊙ L		⊙ R ←
☐	Normal Direct	☐	Normal Indirect	☐	Normal Indirect	☐	Normal Direct
☐	Abnormal Direct	☐	Abnormal Indirect	☐	Abnormal Indirect	☐	Abnormal Direct

  - Nose:_____ ☐NAF
  - Oral cavity: ☐Tarter/Gingivitis (mild / mod / sev),_____ ☐NAF
  - Mandibular lnn.: ☐Enlarged Lt., ☐Enlarged Rt.,_____ ☐NAF

- Neck:_____ ☐NAF
  - Superficial cervical lnn.: ☐Enlarged Lt., ☐Enlarged Rt.,_____ ☐NAF
  - Thyroid:_____ ☐NAF

- Thoracic limb:_____ ☐NAF
  - Foot pads:_____ ☐NAF
  - Knuckling:_____ ☐NAF
  - Axillary lnn. [normally absent]:_____ ☐NAF

- Thorax:_____ ☐NAF

- Abdomen:_____ ☐NAF
  - Mammary chain:_____ ☐NAF
  - Penis/ Testicles/ Vulva:_____ ☐NAF
  - Superficial inguinal lnn. [normally absent]:_____ ☐NAF

- Pelvic limb:_____ ☐NAF
  - Foot pads:_____ ☐NAF
  - Knuckling:_____ ☐NAF
  - Popliteal lnn.: ☐Enlarged Lt., ☐Enlarged Rt.,_____ ☐NAF

- Skin:_____ ☐NAF
- Tail:_____ ☐NAF
- Rectal☞ ☉:_____ ☐NAF

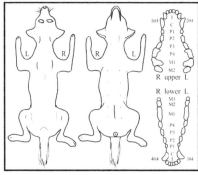
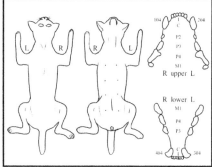

Problems List:

• **Problem #1**:

• **Problem #2**:

• **Problem #3**:

• **Problem #4**:

• **Problem #5**:

Diagnostic Plan	Treatment Plan

Case No._____

Patient	Age	Sex	Breed	Weight
	DOB:	Mn / Mi Fs / Fi	Color:	kg

Owner	Primary Veterinarian	Admit Date/ Time
Name: Phone:	Name: Phone:	Date: Time: AM / PM

• **Presenting Complaint**:_____
_____
_____

• **Medical Hx**:_____
_____
_____

• **When/ where obtained**: Date:_____; ☐Breeder, ☐Shelter, Other:_____

Drug/ Suppl.	Amount	Dose (mg/kg)	Route	Frequency	Date Started

• **Vaccine status – Dog**: ☐Rab ☐Parv ☐Dist ☐Aden; ☐Para ☐Lep ☐Bord ☐Influ ☐Lyme
• **Vaccine status – Cat**: ☐Rab ☐Herp ☐Cali ☐Pan ☐FeLV[kittens]; ☐FIV ☐Chlam ☐Bord
• **Heartworm / Flea & Tick / Intestinal Parasites**:
  ◦ *Last Heartworm Test*: Date:_____, ☐IDK; Test Results: ☐Pos, ☐Neg, ☐IDK
  ◦ *Monthly heartworm preventative*: ☐no ☐yes, Product:_____
  ◦ *Monthly flea & tick preventative*: ☐no ☐yes, Product:_____
  ◦ *Monthly dewormer*: ☐no ☐yes, Product:_____
• **Surgical Hx**: ☐Spay/Neuter; Date:_____; Other:_____
• **Environment**: ☐Indoor, ☐Outdoor, Time spent outdoors/ Other:_____
• **Housemates**: Dogs:_____ Cats:_____ Other:_____
• **Diet**: ☐Wet, ☐Dry; Brand/ Amt.:_____

Appetite	☐Normal, ☐↑, ☐↓
Weight	☐Normal, ☐↑, ☐↓; Past Wt.:_____ kg; Date:_____; Δ:_____
Thirst	☐Normal, ☐↑, ☐↓
Urination	☐Normal, ☐↑, ☐↓, ☐Blood, ☐Strain
Defecation	☐Normal, ☐↑, ☐↓, ☐Blood, ☐Strain, ☐Diarrhea, ☐Mucus
Discharge	☐No, ☐Yes; Onset/ Describe:
Cough/ Sneeze	☐No, ☐Yes; Onset/ Describe:
Vomit	☐No, ☐Yes; Onset/ Describe:
Respiration	☐Normal, ☐↑ Rate, ☐↑ Effort
Energy level	☐Normal, ☐Lethargic, ☐Exercise intolerance

• **Travel Hx**: ☐None, Other:_____
• **Exposure to**: ☐Standing water, ☐Wildlife, ☐Board/daycare, ☐Dog park, ☐Groomer
• **Adverse reactions to food/ meds**: ☐None, Other:_____
• **Can give oral meds**: ☐no ☐yes; Helpful Tricks:_____

Physical Exam – General:

- **Body Weight**:_____kg **Body Condition Score**:_____/9

- **Temperature**:_____°F [*Dog-RI*: 100.9–102.4; *Cat-RI*: 98.1–102.1]

- **Heart**:
  - *Rate*:_____beats/min [Dog-RI: 60–180; Cat-RI: 140–240 (in hospital)]
  - *Rhythm*:   □Regular, □Irregular
  - *Sounds*:   □None, □Split sound, □Gallop, □Murmur, □Muffled
    - *Grade*:   □1–2[soft, only at PMI],   □3–4[moderate, mild radiate],   □5–6[strong radiate, thrill]
    - *Timing*: □Systolic, □Diastolic, □Continuous
    - *PMI*:

	PMI	Over	Anatomic Boundaries
□	Lt. apex	Mitral valve	5th to 6th ICS at level of CCJ
□	Lt. base	Ao + Pul outflow	2nd to 4th ICS above the CCJ
□	Rt. midheart	Tricuspid valve	3rd to 5th ICS near the CCJ
□	Rt. sternal border	Right ventricle	5th to 7th ICS immediately dorsal to the sternum
□	Sternal (cat)	Sternum	In cats, PMI offers very little clinical significance.

  - *Vertebral Heart Size*: Dog = 8.7–10.5; Cat = 6.9–8.1 (from cranial edge of T4)
  - *Innocent Murmur*: Grade 1-2, systolic, left base location, disappear by ~4 months of age, absent clinical signs

- **Pulses**:
  - *Pulse rate*:_____pulses/min
  - *Character*:   □Sync, □Async;   □Normokinetic, □Hyper-, □Hypo-, □Variable

- **Lungs**:
  - *Respiratory rate*:_____breaths/min [*RI*: 16–30]
  - *Depth/Effort*: □Norm, □Pant, □Deep, □Shallow, □↑ Insp effort, □↑ Exp effort
  - *Sounds/Localization*:
    - □Norm BV, □Quiet BV, □Loud BV, □Crack, □Wheez, □Frict, □Muffled
    - □All fields, □Rt cran, □Rt mid, □Rt caud, □Lt cran, □Lt mid, □Lt caud
  - *Tracheal Auscultation/ Palpation*: □Normal, Other:_____

- **Pain Score**:_____ / 5   Localization:_____

- **Mentation**: □BAR   □Confused/   □Drowsy/   □Stuporous   □Coma
                 □QAR   Disoriented   Obtunded   (unresponsive
                 □Dull   unless aroused by
                                                          noxious stimuli)

- **Skin Elasticity**: □Normal skin turgor, □↓ Skin turgor, □Skin tent, □Gelatinous

- **Mucus Membranes**:
  - *CRT*:_____ [*RI*: 1–2; <1 = compensated shock, sepsis, heat stroke; <2 = acute decompensated shock; >2 = late decompensated shock, decreased cardiac output, hypothermia]
  - *Color*:_____ [*RI*: pink; red = compensated shock, sepsis, heat stroke; pale/white = anemia, shock; blue = cyanosis; yellow = hepatic disease, extravascular hemolysis; brown = met-Hb]
  - *Texture*:_____ [*RI*: moist = hydrated; tacky-to-dry = 5–12% dehydrated]

Physical Exam – Systems Checklist:

- Head:_____ ☐NAF
  - ◦ Ears: ☐Debris (mild / mod / sev) (AS / AD / AU), _____ ☐NAF
  - ◦ Eyes:_____ ☐NAF
    - ▪ Retinal:_____ ☐NAF

→ ⚫L	⚫R	⚫L	⚫R ←
☐ Normal Direct	☐ Normal Indirect	☐ Normal Indirect	☐ Normal Direct
☐ Abnormal Direct	☐ Abnormal Indirect	☐ Abnormal Indirect	☐ Abnormal Direct

  - ◦ Nose:_____ ☐NAF
  - ◦ Oral cavity: ☐Tarter/Gingivitis (mild / mod / sev), _____ ☐NAF
  - ◦ Mandibular lnn.: ☐Enlarged Lt., ☐Enlarged Rt., _____ ☐NAF

- Neck:_____ ☐NAF
  - ◦ Superficial cervical lnn.: ☐Enlarged Lt., ☐Enlarged Rt., ____ ☐NAF
  - ◦ Thyroid:_____ ☐NAF

- Thoracic limb:_____ ☐NAF
  - ◦ Foot pads:_____ ☐NAF
  - ◦ Knuckling:_____ ☐NAF
  - ◦ Axillary lnn. [normally absent]:_____ ☐NAF

- Thorax:_____ ☐NAF

- Abdomen:_____ ☐NAF
  - ◦ Mammary chain:_____ ☐NAF
  - ◦ Penis/ Testicles/ Vulva:_____ ☐NAF
  - ◦ Superficial inguinal lnn. [normally absent]:_____ ☐NAF

- Pelvic limb:_____ ☐NAF
  - ◦ Foot pads:_____ ☐NAF
  - ◦ Knuckling:_____ ☐NAF
  - ◦ Popliteal lnn.: ☐Enlarged Lt., ☐Enlarged Rt., _____ ☐NAF

- Skin:_____ ☐NAF
- Tail:_____ ☐NAF
- Rectal☞⊙:_____ ☐NAF

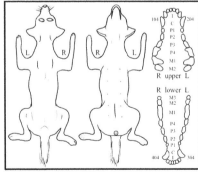

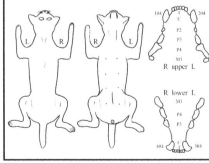

Problems List:

• **Problem #1**:

• **Problem #2**:

• **Problem #3**:

• **Problem #4**:

• **Problem #5**:

Diagnostic Plan	Treatment Plan

Case No._____

Patient	Age	Sex	Breed	Weight
	DOB:	Mn / Mi Fs / Fi	Color:	kg

Owner	Primary Veterinarian	Admit Date/ Time
Name: Phone:	Name: Phone:	Date: Time: AM / PM

• **Presenting Complaint**:_____

_____

• **Medical Hx**:_____

_____

• **When/ where obtained**:   Date:_____; ☐Breeder, ☐Shelter, Other:_____

Drug/ Suppl.	Amount	Dose (mg/kg)	Route	Frequency	Date Started

• **Vaccine status – Dog**: ☐Rab ☐Parv ☐Dist ☐Aden; ☐Para ☐Lep ☐Bord ☐Influ ☐Lyme
• **Vaccine status – Cat**: ☐Rab ☐Herp ☐Cali ☐Pan ☐FeLV[kittens]; ☐FIV ☐Chlam ☐Bord
• **Heartworm / Flea & Tick / Intestinal Parasites**:
  ◦ *Last Heartworm Test*: Date:_____, ☐IDK; Test Results: ☐Pos, ☐Neg, ☐IDK
  ◦ *Monthly heartworm preventative*:   ☐no ☐yes, Product:_____
  ◦ *Monthly flea & tick preventative*:   ☐no ☐yes, Product:_____
  ◦ *Monthly dewormer*:   ☐no ☐yes, Product:_____
• **Surgical Hx**:   ☐Spay/Neuter; Date:_____; Other:_____
• **Environment**: ☐Indoor, ☐Outdoor, Time spent outdoors/ Other:_____
• **Housemates**: Dogs:_____ Cats:_____ Other:_____
• **Diet**: ☐Wet, ☐Dry; Brand/ Amt.:_____

Appetite	☐Normal, ☐↑, ☐↓
Weight	☐Normal, ☐↑, ☐↓; Past Wt.:_____ kg; Date:_____; Δ:_____
Thirst	☐Normal, ☐↑, ☐↓
Urination	☐Normal, ☐↑, ☐↓, ☐Blood, ☐Strain
Defecation	☐Normal, ☐↑, ☐↓, ☐Blood, ☐Strain, ☐Diarrhea, ☐Mucus
Discharge	☐No, ☐Yes; Onset/ Describe:
Cough/ Sneeze	☐No, ☐Yes; Onset/ Describe:
Vomit	☐No, ☐Yes; Onset/ Describe:
Respiration	☐Normal, ☐↑ Rate, ☐↑ Effort
Energy level	☐Normal, ☐Lethargic, ☐Exercise intolerance

• **Travel Hx**: ☐None, Other:_____
• **Exposure to**: ☐Standing water, ☐Wildlife, ☐Board/daycare, ☐Dog park, ☐Groomer
• **Adverse reactions to food/ meds**: ☐None, Other:_____
• **Can give oral meds**: ☐no ☐yes; Helpful Tricks:_____

Physical Exam – General:

- **Body Weight**:_____kg   **Body Condition Score**:_____/9

- **Temperature**:_____°F [*Dog-RI*: 100.9–102.4; *Cat-RI*: 98.1–102.1]

- **Heart**:
  - *Rate*:_____beats/min [Dog-RI: 60–180; Cat-RI: 140–240 (in hospital)]
  - *Rhythm*:   ☐Regular, ☐Irregular
  - *Sounds*:   ☐None, ☐Split sound, ☐Gallop, ☐Murmur, ☐Muffled
    - *Grade*:   ☐1–2[soft, only at PMI],   ☐3–4[moderate, mild radiate],   ☐5–6[strong radiate, thrill]
    - *Timing*: ☐Systolic, ☐Diastolic, ☐Continuous
    - *PMI*:

	PMI	Over	Anatomic Boundaries
☐	Lt. apex	Mitral valve	5th to 6th ICS at level of CCJ
☐	Lt. base	Ao + Pul outflow	2nd to 4th ICS above the CCJ
☐	Rt. midheart	Tricuspid valve	3rd to 5th ICS near the CCJ
☐	Rt. sternal border	Right ventricle	5th to 7th ICS immediately dorsal to the sternum
☐	Sternal (cat)	Sternum	In cats, PMI offers very little clinical significance.

  - • *Vertebral Heart Size*: Dog = 8.7–10.5; Cat = 6.9–8.1 (from cranial edge of T4)
  - • *Innocent Murmur*: Grade 1-2, systolic, left base location, disappear by ~4 months of age, absent clinical signs

- **Pulses**:
  - *Pulse rate*:_____pulses/min
  - *Character*:   ☐Sync, ☐Async;   ☐Normokinetic, ☐Hyper-, ☐Hypo-, ☐Variable

- **Lungs**:
  - *Respiratory rate*:_____breaths/min [*RI*: 16–30]
  - *Depth/Effort*: ☐Norm, ☐Pant, ☐Deep, ☐Shallow, ☐↑ Insp effort, ☐↑ Exp effort
  - *Sounds/Localization*:
    - ☐Norm BV, ☐Quiet BV, ☐Loud BV, ☐Crack, ☐Wheez, ☐Frict, ☐Muffled
    - ☐All fields, ☐Rt cran, ☐Rt mid, ☐Rt caud, ☐Lt cran, ☐Lt mid, ☐Lt caud
  - *Tracheal Auscultation/ Palpation*: ☐Normal, Other:_____

- **Pain Score**:_____ / 5   Localization:_____

- **Mentation**: ☐BAR   ☐Confused/   ☐Drowsy/   ☐Stuporous   ☐Coma
                 ☐QAR   Disoriented   Obtunded   (unresponsive
                 ☐Dull   unless aroused by
                                                                noxious stimuli)

- **Skin Elasticity**: ☐Normal skin turgor, ☐↓ Skin turgor, ☐Skin tent, ☐Gelatinous

- **Mucus Membranes**:
  - *CRT*:_____ [*RI*: 1–2; <1 = compensated shock, sepsis, heat stroke; <2 = acute decompensated shock; >2 = late decompensated shock, decreased cardiac output, hypothermia]
  - *Color*:_____ [*RI*: pink; red = compensated shock, sepsis, heat stroke; pale/white = anemia, shock; blue = cyanosis; yellow = hepatic disease, extravascular hemolysis; brown = met-Hb]
  - *Texture*:_____ [*RI*: moist = hydrated; tacky-to-dry = 5–12% dehydrated]

Physical Exam – Systems Checklist:

- Head:_____ ☐NAF
  - Ears: ☐Debris (mild / mod / sev) (AS / AD / AU),_____ ☐NAF
  - Eyes:_____ ☐NAF
    - Retinal:_____ ☐NAF

☐	Normal Direct	☐	Normal Indirect	☐	Normal Indirect	☐	Normal Direct
☐	Abnormal Direct	☐	Abnormal Indirect	☐	Abnormal Indirect	☐	Abnormal Direct

  - Nose:_____ ☐NAF
  - Oral cavity: ☐Tarter/Gingivitis (mild / mod / sev),_____ ☐NAF
  - Mandibular Inn.: ☐Enlarged Lt., ☐Enlarged Rt.,_____ ☐NAF

- Neck:_____ ☐NAF
  - Superficial cervical Inn.: ☐Enlarged Lt., ☐Enlarged Rt.,_____ ☐NAF
  - Thyroid:_____ ☐NAF

- Thoracic limb:_____ ☐NAF
  - Foot pads:_____ ☐NAF
  - Knuckling:_____ ☐NAF
  - Axillary Inn. [normally absent]:_____ ☐NAF

- Thorax:_____ ☐NAF

- Abdomen:_____ ☐NAF
  - Mammary chain:_____ ☐NAF
  - Penis/ Testicles/ Vulva:_____ ☐NAF
  - Superficial inguinal Inn. [normally absent]:_____ ☐NAF

- Pelvic limb:_____ ☐NAF
  - Foot pads:_____ ☐NAF
  - Knuckling:_____ ☐NAF
  - Popliteal Inn.: ☐Enlarged Lt., ☐Enlarged Rt.,_____ ☐NAF

- Skin:_____ ☐NAF
- Tail:_____ ☐NAF
- Rectal☞☉:_____ ☐NAF

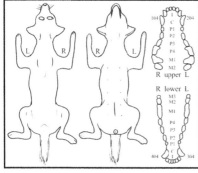

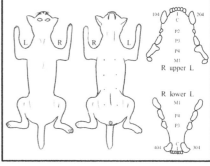

<u>**Problems List**</u>:

• **Problem #1**:

• **Problem #2**:

• **Problem #3**:

• **Problem #4**:

• **Problem #5**:

Diagnostic Plan	Treatment Plan

Case No._____

Patient	Age	Sex	Breed	Weight
	DOB:	Mn / Mi Fs / Fi	Color:	kg

Owner	Primary Veterinarian	Admit Date/ Time
Name: Phone:	Name: Phone:	Date: Time: AM / PM

• **Presenting Complaint**:_____

_____

• **Medical Hx**:_____

_____

• **When/ where obtained**: Date:_____; ☐Breeder, ☐Shelter, Other:_____

Drug/ Suppl.	Amount	Dose (mg/kg)	Route	Frequency	Date Started

• **Vaccine status – Dog**: ☐Rab ☐Parv ☐Dist ☐Aden; ☐Para ☐Lep ☐Bord ☐Influ ☐Lyme
• **Vaccine status – Cat**: ☐Rab ☐Herp ☐Cali ☐Pan ☐FeLV[kittens]; ☐FIV ☐Chlam ☐Bord
• **Heartworm / Flea & Tick / Intestinal Parasites**:
  ◦ *Last Heartworm Test*: Date:_____, ☐IDK; Test Results: ☐Pos, ☐Neg, ☐IDK
  ◦ *Monthly heartworm preventative*: ☐no ☐yes, Product:_____
  ◦ *Monthly flea & tick preventative*: ☐no ☐yes, Product:_____
  ◦ *Monthly dewormer*: ☐no ☐yes, Product:_____
• **Surgical Hx**: ☐Spay/Neuter; Date:_____; Other:_____
• **Environment**: ☐Indoor, ☐Outdoor, Time spent outdoors/ Other:_____
• **Housemates**: Dogs:_____ Cats:_____ Other:_____
• **Diet**: ☐Wet, ☐Dry; Brand/ Amt.:_____

Appetite	☐Normal, ☐↑, ☐↓
Weight	☐Normal, ☐↑, ☐↓; Past Wt.:_____ kg; Date:_____; Δ:_____
Thirst	☐Normal, ☐↑, ☐↓
Urination	☐Normal, ☐↑, ☐↓, ☐Blood, ☐Strain
Defecation	☐Normal, ☐↑, ☐↓, ☐Blood, ☐Strain, ☐Diarrhea, ☐Mucus
Discharge	☐No, ☐Yes; Onset/ Describe:
Cough/ Sneeze	☐No, ☐Yes; Onset/ Describe:
Vomit	☐No, ☐Yes; Onset/ Describe:
Respiration	☐Normal, ☐↑ Rate, ☐↑ Effort
Energy level	☐Normal, ☐Lethargic, ☐Exercise intolerance

• **Travel Hx**: ☐None, Other:_____
• **Exposure to**: ☐Standing water, ☐Wildlife, ☐Board/daycare, ☐Dog park, ☐Groomer
• **Adverse reactions to food/ meds**: ☐None, Other:_____
• **Can give oral meds**: ☐no ☐yes; Helpful Tricks:_____

Physical Exam – General:

- **Body Weight**:_____kg   **Body Condition Score**:_____/9

- **Temperature**:_____°F [*Dog-RI*: 100.9–102.4; *Cat-RI*: 98.1–102.1]

- **Heart**:
  - *Rate*:_____beats/min [Dog-RI: 60–180; Cat-RI: 140–240 (in hospital)]
  - *Rhythm*: ☐Regular, ☐Irregular
  - *Sounds*: ☐None, ☐Split sound, ☐Gallop, ☐Murmur, ☐Muffled
    - *Grade*: ☐1–2[soft, only at PMI], ☐3–4[moderate, mild radiate], ☐5–6[strong radiate, thrill]
    - *Timing*: ☐Systolic, ☐Diastolic, ☐Continuous
    - *PMI*:

	PMI	Over	Anatomic Boundaries
☐	Lt. apex	Mitral valve	5th to 6th ICS at level of CCJ
☐	Lt. base	Ao + Pul outflow	2nd to 4th ICS above the CCJ
☐	Rt. midheart	Tricuspid valve	3rd to 5th ICS near the CCJ
☐	Rt. sternal border	Right ventricle	5th to 7th ICS immediately dorsal to the sternum
☐	Sternal (cat)	Sternum	In cats, PMI offers very little clinical significance.

-    *Vertebral Heart Size*: Dog = 8.7–10.5; Cat = 6.9–8.1 (from cranial edge of T4)
-    *Innocent Murmur*: Grade 1-2, systolic, left base location, disappear by ~4 months of age, absent clinical signs

- **Pulses**:
  - *Pulse rate*:_____pulses/min
  - *Character*: ☐Sync, ☐Async; ☐Normokinetic, ☐Hyper-, ☐Hypo-, ☐Variable

- **Lungs**:
  - *Respiratory rate*:_____breaths/min [*RI*: 16–30]
  - *Depth/Effort*: ☐Norm, ☐Pant, ☐Deep, ☐Shallow, ☐↑ Insp effort, ☐↑ Exp effort
  - *Sounds/Localization*:
    - ☐Norm BV, ☐Quiet BV, ☐Loud BV, ☐Crack, ☐Wheez, ☐Frict, ☐Muffled
    - ☐All fields, ☐Rt cran, ☐Rt mid, ☐Rt caud, ☐Lt cran, ☐Lt mid, ☐Lt caud
  - *Tracheal Auscultation/ Palpation*: ☐Normal, Other:_____

- **Pain Score**:_____ / 5   Localization:_____

- **Mentation**: ☐BAR   ☐Confused/   ☐Drowsy/   ☐Stuporous   ☐Coma
             ☐QAR   Disoriented   Obtunded   (unresponsive
             ☐Dull   unless aroused by
                                                noxious stimuli)

- **Skin Elasticity**: ☐Normal skin turgor, ☐↓ Skin turgor, ☐Skin tent, ☐Gelatinous

- **Mucus Membranes**:
  - *CRT*:_____ [*RI*: 1–2; <1 = compensated shock, sepsis, heat stroke; <2 = acute decompensated shock; >2 = late decompensated shock, decreased cardiac output, hypothermia]
  - *Color*:_____ [*RI*: pink; red = compensated shock, sepsis, heat stroke; pale/white = anemia, shock; blue = cyanosis; yellow = hepatic disease, extravascular hemolysis; brown = met-Hb]
  - *Texture*:_____ [*RI*: moist = hydrated; tacky-to-dry = 5–12% dehydrated]

<u>Physical Exam – Systems Checklist</u>:

- Head:_____ ☐NAF
  - ◦ Ears: ☐Debris (mild / mod / sev) (AS / AD / AU),_____ ☐NAF
  - ◦ Eyes:_____ ☐NAF
    - ▪ Retinal:_____ ☐NAF

→ Ⓛ		Ⓡ		Ⓛ		Ⓡ ←	
☐	Normal Direct	☐	Normal Indirect	☐	Normal Indirect	☐	Normal Direct
☐	Abnormal Direct	☐	Abnormal Indirect	☐	Abnormal Indirect	☐	Abnormal Direct

  - ◦ Nose:_____ ☐NAF
  - ◦ Oral cavity: ☐Tarter/Gingivitis (mild / mod / sev),_____ ☐NAF
  - ◦ Mandibular lnn.: ☐Enlarged Lt., ☐Enlarged Rt.,_____ ☐NAF

- Neck:_____ ☐NAF
  - ◦ Superficial cervical lnn.: ☐Enlarged Lt., ☐Enlarged Rt.,_____ ☐NAF
  - ◦ Thyroid:_____ ☐NAF

- Thoracic limb:_____ ☐NAF
  - ◦ Foot pads:_____ ☐NAF
  - ◦ Knuckling:_____ ☐NAF
  - ◦ Axillary lnn. [normally absent]:_____ ☐NAF

- Thorax:_____ ☐NAF

- Abdomen:_____ ☐NAF
  - ◦ Mammary chain:_____ ☐NAF
  - ◦ Penis/ Testicles/ Vulva:_____ ☐NAF
  - ◦ Superficial inguinal lnn. [normally absent]:_____ ☐NAF

- Pelvic limb:_____ ☐NAF
  - ◦ Foot pads:_____ ☐NAF
  - ◦ Knuckling:_____ ☐NAF
  - ◦ Popliteal lnn.: ☐Enlarged Lt., ☐Enlarged Rt.,_____ ☐NAF

- Skin:_____ ☐NAF
- Tail:_____ ☐NAF
- Rectal☞☉:_____ ☐NAF

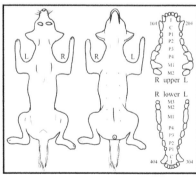

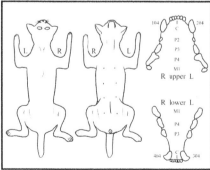

Problems List:

• **Problem #1**:

• **Problem #2**:

• **Problem #3**:

• **Problem #4**:

• **Problem #5**:

Diagnostic Plan	Treatment Plan

Case No._____

Patient	Age	Sex	Breed	Weight
	DOB:	Mn / Mi Fs / Fi	Color:	kg

Owner	Primary Veterinarian	Admit Date/ Time
Name: Phone:	Name: Phone:	Date: Time: AM / PM

• **Presenting Complaint**:_____

_____

• **Medical Hx**:_____

_____

• **When/ where obtained**: Date:_____; ☐Breeder, ☐Shelter, Other:_____

Drug/ Suppl.	Amount	Dose (mg/kg)	Route	Frequency	Date Started

• **Vaccine status – Dog**: ☐Rab ☐Parv ☐Dist ☐Aden; ☐Para ☐Lep ☐Bord ☐Influ ☐Lyme
• **Vaccine status – Cat**: ☐Rab ☐Herp ☐Cali ☐Pan ☐FeLV[kittens]; ☐FIV ☐Chlam ☐Bord
• **Heartworm / Flea & Tick / Intestinal Parasites**:
   ◦ *Last Heartworm Test*: Date:_____, ☐IDK; Test Results: ☐Pos, ☐Neg, ☐IDK
   ◦ *Monthly heartworm preventative*: ☐no ☐yes, Product:_____
   ◦ *Monthly flea & tick preventative*: ☐no ☐yes, Product:_____
   ◦ *Monthly dewormer*:   ☐no ☐yes, Product:_____
• **Surgical Hx**: ☐Spay/Neuter; Date:_____; Other:_____
• **Environment**: ☐Indoor, ☐Outdoor, Time spent outdoors/ Other:_____
• **Housemates**: Dogs:_____ Cats:_____ Other:_____
• **Diet**: ☐Wet, ☐Dry; Brand/ Amt.:_____

Appetite	☐Normal, ☐↑, ☐↓
Weight	☐Normal, ☐↑, ☐↓; Past Wt.:_____ kg; Date:_____; Δ:_____
Thirst	☐Normal, ☐↑, ☐↓
Urination	☐Normal, ☐↑, ☐↓, ☐Blood, ☐Strain
Defecation	☐Normal, ☐↑, ☐↓, ☐Blood, ☐Strain, ☐Diarrhea, ☐Mucus
Discharge	☐No, ☐Yes; Onset/ Describe:
Cough/ Sneeze	☐No, ☐Yes; Onset/ Describe:
Vomit	☐No, ☐Yes; Onset/ Describe:
Respiration	☐Normal, ☐↑ Rate, ☐↑ Effort
Energy level	☐Normal, ☐Lethargic, ☐Exercise intolerance

• **Travel Hx**: ☐None, Other:_____
• **Exposure to**: ☐Standing water, ☐Wildlife, ☐Board/daycare, ☐Dog park, ☐Groomer
• **Adverse reactions to food/ meds**: ☐None, Other:_____
• **Can give oral meds**: ☐no ☐yes; Helpful Tricks:_____

Physical Exam – General:

- **Body Weight**: _____ kg   **Body Condition Score**: _____ /9

- **Temperature**: _____ °F [*Dog-RI*: 100.9–102.4; *Cat-RI*: 98.1–102.1]

- **Heart**:
  - *Rate*: _____ beats/min [Dog-RI: 60–180; Cat-RI: 140–240 (in hospital)]
  - *Rhythm*:   □Regular, □Irregular
  - *Sounds*:   □None, □Split sound, □Gallop, □Murmur, □Muffled
    - *Grade*:   □1–2[soft, only at PMI],   □3–4[moderate, mild radiate],   □5–6[strong radiate, thrill]
    - *Timing*: □Systolic, □Diastolic, □Continuous
    - *PMI*:

	PMI	Over	Anatomic Boundaries
□	Lt. apex	Mitral valve	5th to 6th ICS at level of CCJ
□	Lt. base	Ao + Pul outflow	2nd to 4th ICS above the CCJ
□	Rt. midheart	Tricuspid valve	3rd to 5th ICS near the CCJ
□	Rt. sternal border	Right ventricle	5th to 7th ICS immediately dorsal to the sternum
□	Sternal (cat)	Sternum	In cats, PMI offers very little clinical significance.

- *Vertebral Heart Size*: Dog = 8.7–10.5; Cat = 6.9–8.1 (from cranial edge of T4)
- *Innocent Murmur*: Grade 1-2, systolic, left base location, disappear by ~4 months of age, absent clinical signs

- **Pulses**:
  - *Pulse rate*: _____ pulses/min
  - *Character*:   □Sync, □Async;   □Normokinetic, □Hyper-, □Hypo-, □Variable

- **Lungs**:
  - *Respiratory rate*: _____ breaths/min [*RI*: 16–30]
  - *Depth/Effort*: □Norm, □Pant, □Deep, □Shallow, □↑ Insp effort, □↑ Exp effort
  - *Sounds/Localization*:
    - □Norm BV, □Quiet BV, □Loud BV, □Crack, □Wheez, □Frict, □Muffled
    - □All fields, □Rt cran, □Rt mid, □Rt caud, □Lt cran, □Lt mid, □Lt caud
  - *Tracheal Auscultation/ Palpation*: □Normal, Other: _____

- **Pain Score**: _____ / 5   Localization: _____

- **Mentation**: □BAR   □Confused/   □Drowsy/   □Stuporous   □Coma
  □QAR   Disoriented   Obtunded   (unresponsive
  □Dull   unless aroused by
  noxious stimuli)

- **Skin Elasticity**: □Normal skin turgor, □↓ Skin turgor, □Skin tent, □Gelatinous

- **Mucus Membranes**:
  - *CRT*: _____ [*RI*: 1–2; <1 = compensated shock, sepsis, heat stroke; <2 = acute decompensated shock; >2 = late decompensated shock, decreased cardiac output, hypothermia]
  - *Color*: _____ [*RI*: pink; red = compensated shock, sepsis, heat stroke; pale/white = anemia, shock; blue = cyanosis; yellow = hepatic disease, extravascular hemolysis; brown = met-Hb]
  - *Texture*: _____ [*RI*: moist = hydrated; tacky-to-dry = 5–12% dehydrated]

Physical Exam – Systems Checklist:

- Head:_____ ☐NAF
  - Ears: ☐Debris (mild / mod / sev) (AS / AD / AU), _____ ☐NAF
  - Eyes:_____ ☐NAF
    - Retinal:_____ ☐NAF

→ **Ⓛ**		**Ⓡ**		**Ⓛ**		**Ⓡ** ←	
☐	Normal Direct	☐	Normal Indirect	☐	Normal Indirect	☐	Normal Direct
☐	Abnormal Direct	☐	Abnormal Indirect	☐	Abnormal Indirect	☐	Abnormal Direct

  - Nose:_____ ☐NAF
  - Oral cavity: ☐Tarter/Gingivitis (mild / mod / sev), _____ ☐NAF
  - Mandibular lnn.: ☐Enlarged Lt., ☐Enlarged Rt., _____ ☐NAF

- Neck:_____ ☐NAF
  - Superficial cervical lnn.: ☐Enlarged Lt., ☐Enlarged Rt., _____ ☐NAF
  - Thyroid:_____ ☐NAF

- Thoracic limb:_____ ☐NAF
  - Foot pads:_____ ☐NAF
  - Knuckling:_____ ☐NAF
  - Axillary lnn. [normally absent]:_____ ☐NAF

- Thorax:_____ ☐NAF

- Abdomen:_____ ☐NAF
  - Mammary chain:_____ ☐NAF
  - Penis/ Testicles/ Vulva:_____ ☐NAF
  - Superficial inguinal lnn. [normally absent]:_____ ☐NAF

- Pelvic limb:_____ ☐NAF
  - Foot pads:_____ ☐NAF
  - Knuckling:_____ ☐NAF
  - Popliteal lnn.: ☐Enlarged Lt., ☐Enlarged Rt., _____ ☐NAF

- Skin:_____ ☐NAF
- Tail:_____ ☐NAF
- Rectal☞☉:_____ ☐NAF

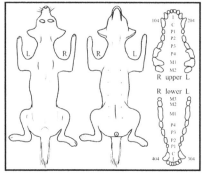
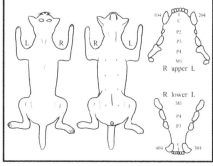

Problems List:

• Problem #1:

• Problem #2:

• Problem #3:

• Problem #4:

• Problem #5:

Diagnostic Plan	Treatment Plan

[Intentionally Left Blank]

Orthopedic, Neurologic, and Optic Exams

Orthopedic Examination:

Patient:_____   **Date**:_____

- General Appearance:
  - Disposition:_____
  - Weight status:_____
  - Limb alignment:_____
  - Positive (failed) sit test: ☐yes, ☐no _____
  - Overt:
    - Lameness: _____ ☐NAF
    - Asym. joint swellings:_____ ☐NAF
    - Asym. soft tis. swellings:_____ ☐NAF
    - Muscle atrophy:_____ ☐NAF

- Gait evaluation:
  [*Abnormality examples*: shortened stride, dragging of the toe-nails, toeing-in or toeing-out, limb circumduction, long-strided gait, meniscal click, head bob, hip sway, *stumbling, *ataxia, *tetraparesis, or *paraparesis (*findings that suggest neuro)]
  - Abnormalities at walk: ☐None, Other:_____
  - Abnormalities at trot: ☐None, Other:_____

- Standing Palpation:
  [*Abnormality examples*: joint effusion or thickening (medial buttress), heat, malalignment of bony landmarks, crepitus, atrophy]
  - *Thoracic Limb*:
    - Acromion:_____ ☐NAF
    - Spine of scapula:_____ ☐NAF
    - G. tubercle of hum.:_____ ☐NAF
    - Hum. Epicondyles:_____ ☐NAF
    - Olecranon:_____ ☐NAF
    - Acc. carpal bn.:_____ ☐NAF
    - Conscious proprioception:_____ ☐NAF

  - *Pelvic Limb*:
    - Normal triangular orientation of ilial wing, tuber ischii, and greater trochanter: ☐yes, ☐no [Linear orientation of landmarks indicates craniodorsal hip luxation.]
    - Iliac crest:_____ ☐NAF
    - Ischiatic tuberosity:_____ ☐NAF
    - G. trochanter of fem.:_____ ☐NAF
    - Quadriceps m.:_____ ☐NAF
    - Patella/ patellar ten.:_____ ☐NAF
      - Able to define cranial 2/3 of patellar tendon: ☐yes, ☐no _____
      - Patellar luxation: ☐yes, ☐no _____
        ☐1(In-Out-In),   ☐2(In-Out-Out),   ☐3(Out-In-Out),   ☐4(Out-Out-Out)
    - Tibial tuberosity:_____ ☐NAF
    - Hamstring mm.:_____ ☐NAF
    - Femoral condyles:_____ ☐NAF
    - Distal tibia:_____ ☐NAF
    - Achilles tendon:_____ ☐NAF
    - Tuber calcaneous:_____ ☐NAF
    - Tarsal joint:_____ ☐NAF
    - Conscious proprioception:_____ ☐NAF

  - *Vertebral Column*:
    - Spinal hyperesthesia: ☐yes, ☐no _____
    - Tail pain: ☐yes, ☐no _____
    - Sacroiliac jt. pain: ☐yes, ☐no _____

- Recumbent Palpation:

  [Abnormality examples: CREPI – crepitus, decreased range-of-motion, effusion, pain, instability]
  - *Right Thoracic Limb*:
    - Footpads/ interdigital webs: _____ ☐NAF
    - Flex/ extend digital joints: _____ ☐NAF
    - Flex/ extend/ varus/ valgus of carpal joints: _____ ☐NAF
    - Flex/ extend elbow joint: _____ ☐NAF
    - Int./ ext. rotation of elbow w/ med. digital pres.: _____ ☐NAF
    - Flex/ extend shoulder joint: _____ ☐NAF

  - *Left Thoracic Limb*:
    - Footpads/ interdigital webs: _____ ☐NAF
    - Flex/ extend digital joints: _____ ☐NAF
    - Flex/ extend/ varus/ valgus of carpal joints: _____ ☐NAF
    - Flex/ extend elbow joint: _____ ☐NAF
    - Int./ ext. rotation of elbow w/ med. digital pres.: _____ ☐NAF
    - Flex/ extend shoulder joint: _____ ☐NAF

  - *Right Pelvic Limb*:
    - Footpads/ interdigital webs: _____ ☐NAF
    - Flex/ extend digital joints: _____ ☐NAF
    - Flex/ extend/ varus/ valgus of tarsal joints: _____ ☐NAF
    - Palpation of achilles tendon:
      - During flexion of tarsal and stifle joints: _____ ☐NAF
      - During extension of tarsal and stifle joints: _____ ☐NAF
    - Palpation of stifle joint:
      - Patellar luxation: ☐yes, ☐no _____
      - Cranial drawer: ☐yes, ☐no _____
      - Cranial tibial thrust: ☐yes, ☐no _____

  - *Left Pelvic Limb*:
    - Footpads/ interdigital webs: _____ ☐NAF
    - Flex/ extend digital joints: _____ ☐NAF
    - Flex/ extend/ varus/ valgus of tarsal joints: _____ ☐NAF
    - Palpation of achilles tendon:
      - During flexion of tarsal and stifle joints: _____ ☐NAF
      - During extension of tarsal and stifle joints: _____ ☐NAF
    - Palpation of stifle joint:
      - Patellar luxation: ☐yes, ☐no _____
      - Cranial drawer: ☐yes, ☐no _____
      - Cranial tibial thrust: ☐yes, ☐no _____

  - *Right Hip & Pelvis*:
    - Flexion/ extension of hip joint: _____ ☐NAF
    - ± Abduction of hip joint: _____ ☐NAF
    - Ortolani sign: ☐yes, ☐no _____

  - *Left Hip & Pelvis*:
    - Flexion/ extension of hip joint: _____ ☐NAF
    - ± Abduction of hip joint: _____ ☐NAF
    - Ortolani sign: ☐yes, ☐no _____

Orthopedic Examination:

Patient:_____   **Date**:_____

- **General Appearance**:
  - Disposition:_____
  - Weight status:_____
  - Limb alignment:_____
  - Positive (failed) sit test: ☐yes, ☐no _____
  - Overt:
    - Lameness: _____ ☐NAF
    - Asym. joint swellings:_____ ☐NAF
    - Asym. soft tis. swellings:_____ ☐NAF
    - Muscle atrophy:_____ ☐NAF

- **Gait evaluation**:
  [*Abnormality examples*: shortened stride, dragging of the toe-nails, toeing-in or toeing-out, limb circumduction, long-strided gait, meniscal click, head bob, hip sway, *stumbling, *ataxia, *tetraparesis, or *paraparesis (*findings that suggest neuro)]
  - Abnormalities at walk: ☐None, Other:_____
  - Abnormalities at trot: ☐None, Other:_____

- **Standing Palpation**:
  [*Abnormality examples*: joint effusion or thickening (medial buttress), heat, malalignment of bony landmarks, crepitus, atrophy]
  - *Thoracic Limb*:
    - Acromion:_____ ☐NAF
    - Spine of scapula:_____ ☐NAF
    - G. tubercle of hum.:_____ ☐NAF
    - Hum. Epicondyles:_____ ☐NAF
    - Olecranon:_____ ☐NAF
    - Acc. carpal bn.:_____ ☐NAF
    - Conscious proprioception:_____ ☐NAF

  - *Pelvic Limb*:
    - Normal triangular orientation of ilial wing, tuber ischii, and greater trochanter: ☐yes, ☐no [Linear orientation of landmarks indicates craniodorsal hip luxation.]
    - Iliac crest:_____ ☐NAF
    - Ischiatic tuberosity:_____ ☐NAF
    - G. trochanter of fem.:_____ ☐NAF
    - Quadriceps m.:_____ ☐NAF
    - Patella/ patellar ten.:_____ ☐NAF
      - Able to define cranial 2/3 of patellar tendon: ☐yes, ☐no _____
      - Patellar luxation: ☐yes, ☐no _____
        ☐1(In-Out-In),   ☐2(In-Out-Out),   ☐3(Out-In-Out),   ☐4(Out-Out-Out)
    - Tibial tuberosity:_____ ☐NAF
    - Hamstring mm.:_____ ☐NAF
    - Femoral condyles:_____ ☐NAF
    - Distal tibia:_____ ☐NAF
    - Achilles tendon:_____ ☐NAF
    - Tuber calcaneous:_____ ☐NAF
    - Tarsal joint:_____ ☐NAF
    - Conscious proprioception:_____ ☐NAF

  - *Vertebral Column*:
    - Spinal hyperesthesia: ☐yes, ☐no _____
    - Tail pain: ☐yes, ☐no _____
    - Sacroiliac jt. pain: ☐yes, ☐no _____

- Recumbent Palpation:
  [*Abnormality examples*: CREPI – crepitus, decreased range-of-motion, effusion, pain, instability]
  - *Right Thoracic Limb*:
    - Footpads/ interdigital webs:_____ ☐NAF
    - Flex/ extend digital joints:_____ ☐NAF
    - Flex/ extend/ varus/ valgus of carpal joints:_____ ☐NAF
    - Flex/ extend elbow joint:_____ ☐NAF
    - Int./ ext. rotation of elbow w/ med. digital pres.:_____ ☐NAF
    - Flex/ extend shoulder joint:_____ ☐NAF

  - *Left Thoracic Limb*:
    - Footpads/ interdigital webs:_____ ☐NAF
    - Flex/ extend digital joints:_____ ☐NAF
    - Flex/ extend/ varus/ valgus of carpal joints:_____ ☐NAF
    - Flex/ extend elbow joint:_____ ☐NAF
    - Int./ ext. rotation of elbow w/ med. digital pres.:_____ ☐NAF
    - Flex/ extend shoulder joint:_____ ☐NAF

  - *Right Pelvic Limb*:
    - Footpads/ interdigital webs:_____ ☐NAF
    - Flex/ extend digital joints:_____ ☐NAF
    - Flex/ extend/ varus/ valgus of tarsal joints:_____ ☐NAF
    - Palpation of achilles tendon:
      - During flexion of tarsal and stifle joints:_____ ☐NAF
      - During extension of tarsal and stifle joints:_____ ☐NAF
    - Palpation of stifle joint:
      - Patellar luxation: ☐yes, ☐no _____
      - Cranial drawer: ☐yes, ☐no _____
      - Cranial tibial thrust: ☐yes, ☐no _____

  - *Left Pelvic Limb*:
    - Footpads/ interdigital webs:_____ ☐NAF
    - Flex/ extend digital joints:_____ ☐NAF
    - Flex/ extend/ varus/ valgus of tarsal joints:_____ ☐NAF
    - Palpation of achilles tendon:
      - During flexion of tarsal and stifle joints:_____ ☐NAF
      - During extension of tarsal and stifle joints:_____ ☐NAF
    - Palpation of stifle joint:
      - Patellar luxation: ☐yes, ☐no _____
      - Cranial drawer: ☐yes, ☐no _____
      - Cranial tibial thrust: ☐yes, ☐no _____

  - *Right Hip & Pelvis*:
    - Flexion/ extension of hip joint:_____ ☐NAF
    - ± Abduction of hip joint:_____ ☐NAF
    - Ortolani sign: ☐yes, ☐no _____

  - *Left Hip & Pelvis*:
    - Flexion/ extension of hip joint:_____ ☐NAF
    - ± Abduction of hip joint:_____ ☐NAF
    - Ortolani sign: ☐yes, ☐no _____

Orthopedic Examination:

Patient:_____   **Date:**_____

- General Appearance:
  - ○ Disposition:_____
  - ○ Weight status:_____
  - ○ Limb alignment:_____
  - ○ Positive (failed) sit test: □yes, □no _____
  - ○ Overt:
    - ▪ Lameness: _____ □NAF
    - ▪ Asym. joint swellings:_____ □NAF
    - ▪ Asym. soft tis. swellings:_____ □NAF
    - ▪ Muscle atrophy:_____ □NAF

- Gait evaluation:
  [*Abnormality examples*: shortened stride, dragging of the toe-nails, toeing-in or toeing-out, limb circumduction, long-strided gait, meniscal click, head bob, hip sway, *stumbling, *ataxia, *tetraparesis, or *paraparesis (*findings that suggest neuro)]
  - ○ Abnormalities at walk: □None, Other:_____
  - ○ Abnormalities at trot: □None, Other:_____

- Standing Palpation:
  [*Abnormality examples*: joint effusion or thickening (medial buttress), heat, malalignment of bony landmarks, crepitus, atrophy]
  - ○ *Thoracic Limb*:
    - ▪ Acromion:_____ □NAF
    - ▪ Spine of scapula:_____ □NAF
    - ▪ G. tubercle of hum.:_____ □NAF
    - ▪ Hum. Epicondyles:_____ □NAF
    - ▪ Olecranon:_____ □NAF
    - ▪ Acc. carpal bn.:_____ □NAF
    - ▪ Conscious proprioception:_____ □NAF

  - ○ *Pelvic Limb*:
    - ▪ Normal triangular orientation of ilial wing, tuber ischii, and greater trochanter: □yes, □no [Linear orientation of landmarks indicates craniodorsal hip luxation.]
    - ▪ Iliac crest:_____ □NAF
    - ▪ Ischiatic tuberosity:_____ □NAF
    - ▪ G. trochanter of fem.:_____ □NAF
    - ▪ Quadriceps m.:_____ □NAF
    - ▪ Patella/ patellar ten.:_____ □NAF
      - • Able to define cranial 2/3 of patellar tendon: □yes, □no _____
      - • Patellar luxation: □yes, □no _____
        □1(In-Out-In), □2(In-Out-Out), □3(Out-In-Out), □4(Out-Out-Out)
    - ▪ Tibial tuberosity:_____ □NAF
    - ▪ Hamstring mm.:_____ □NAF
    - ▪ Femoral condyles:_____ □NAF
    - ▪ Distal tibia:_____ □NAF
    - ▪ Achilles tendon:_____ □NAF
    - ▪ Tuber calcaneous:_____ □NAF
    - ▪ Tarsal joint:_____ □NAF
    - ▪ Conscious proprioception:_____ □NAF

  - ○ *Vertebral Column*:
    - ▪ Spinal hyperesthesia: □yes, □no _____
    - ▪ Tail pain: □yes, □no _____
    - ▪ Sacroiliac jt. pain: □yes, □no _____

- Recumbent Palpation:
  [*Abnormality examples*: CREPI – crepitus, decreased range-of-motion, effusion, pain, instability]
  - *Right Thoracic Limb*:
    - Footpads/ interdigital webs:_____ ☐NAF
    - Flex/ extend digital joints:_____ ☐NAF
    - Flex/ extend/ varus/ valgus of carpal joints:_____ ☐NAF
    - Flex/ extend elbow joint:_____ ☐NAF
    - Int./ ext. rotation of elbow w/ med. digital pres.:_____ ☐NAF
    - Flex/ extend shoulder joint:_____ ☐NAF

  - *Left Thoracic Limb*:
    - Footpads/ interdigital webs:_____ ☐NAF
    - Flex/ extend digital joints:_____ ☐NAF
    - Flex/ extend/ varus/ valgus of carpal joints:_____ ☐NAF
    - Flex/ extend elbow joint:_____ ☐NAF
    - Int./ ext. rotation of elbow w/ med. digital pres.:_____ ☐NAF
    - Flex/ extend shoulder joint:_____ ☐NAF

  - *Right Pelvic Limb*:
    - Footpads/ interdigital webs:_____ ☐NAF
    - Flex/ extend digital joints:_____ ☐NAF
    - Flex/ extend/ varus/ valgus of tarsal joints:_____ ☐NAF
    - Palpation of achilles tendon:
      - During flexion of tarsal and stifle joints:_____ ☐NAF
      - During extension of tarsal and stifle joints:_____ ☐NAF
    - Palpation of stifle joint:
      - Patellar luxation: ☐yes, ☐no _____
      - Cranial drawer: ☐yes, ☐no _____
      - Cranial tibial thrust: ☐yes, ☐no _____

  - *Left Pelvic Limb*:
    - Footpads/ interdigital webs:_____ ☐NAF
    - Flex/ extend digital joints:_____ ☐NAF
    - Flex/ extend/ varus/ valgus of tarsal joints:_____ ☐NAF
    - Palpation of achilles tendon:
      - During flexion of tarsal and stifle joints:_____ ☐NAF
      - During extension of tarsal and stifle joints:_____ ☐NAF
    - Palpation of stifle joint:
      - Patellar luxation: ☐yes, ☐no _____
      - Cranial drawer: ☐yes, ☐no _____
      - Cranial tibial thrust: ☐yes, ☐no _____

  - *Right Hip & Pelvis*:
    - Flexion/ extension of hip joint:_____ ☐NAF
    - ± Abduction of hip joint:_____ ☐NAF
    - Ortolani sign: ☐yes, ☐no _____

  - *Left Hip & Pelvis*:
    - Flexion/ extension of hip joint:_____ ☐NAF
    - ± Abduction of hip joint:_____ ☐NAF
    - Ortolani sign: ☐yes, ☐no _____

Neurological Examination

Patient: _____   **Date**: _____

- **Neurological History**:
    - *Onset Date*: _____
    - *Duration*: _____
    - *Progression*: (*peracute / acute / chronic / progressive / static*) _____

- **Previous Treatments**:

Drug	Amount	Dose (mg/kg)	Route	Frequency	Duration

- *Mental Status*:

Alert (conscious; responds to sensory stimuli)	Obtunded (↓ interaction w/ environment; slow response to verbal stimuli)	Stupor (unresponsive unless aroused by noxious stimuli)	Coma (complete unresponsiveness to any stimuli)

- *Posture*:

Normal	Head Tilt (L / R)	Tremor	Falling	Circling (Tight / Wide) (L / R)
Schiff-Sherrington (rigid extension of forelimbs w/out forelimb paresis or ataxia)	Opisthotonus (backward arching of head, neck, and spine)	Decerebrate (opisthotonus + rigid extension of all limbs + stupor or coma)	Decerebellate (opisthotonus + rigid extension of fore-limbs + hip flexion + normal mentation)	

- *Gait*:   *Affected Limb(s)*:

Ambulatory (able to stand and walk 10 steps unaided)		Non-ambulatory (unable to stand and walk 10 steps unaided)		
Normal	Paraparesis	Paraplegia	Tetraparesis	Tetraplegia
Monoparesis	Monoplegia	Hemiparesis	Hemiplegia	
Proprioceptive Ataxia		Cerebellar Ataxia		Vestib. Ataxia

- *Motor*:   Yes (voluntary movement)   No (absence of voluntary movement)

- *Urination*:   Yes (voluntary urination)   No (absence of voluntary urination)

(0=absent, 1=hypo, 2=normal)

L	Knuckling	R
	Front	
	Rear	

L	Hopping	R
	Front	
	Rear	

L	Ext. Post. Thrust	R
	Rear	

L	Wheelbarrowing	R
	Visual	
	Non-visual	

(0=absent, 1=hypo, 2=norm, 3=hyper, 4=clonus)

L	Nerve Function	R
	Biceps (C6-C8)	
	Triceps (C7-T1)	
	Extensor Carpi (C7-T1)	
	Withdrawal Forelimb (C6-T2)	
	Patellar (L4-L6)	
	Cranial Tibial (L6-L7)	
	Gastrocnemius (L6-S1)	
	Withdrawal Hindlimb (L5-S1)	
	Perineal (S1-S2)	
	Panniculus	
	Cross Extensor	
	Tail Tone	
	Anal Tone	

Neuroanatomical Localization
Generalized neuromuscular, Spinal cord (C1-C5),   Spinal cord (C6-T2), Spinal cord (T3-L3),   Spinal cord (L4-Cd5), Caudal brainstem,   Cerebellum,   Forebrain, Multifocal,   Diffuse

(0=absent, 1=hypo, 2=normal)

L	Nerve Function	R
	Vision & Menace (2)	
	Pupil Size (2, 3)	
	Direct PLR (2, 3)	
	Indirect PLR (2, 3)	
	Palpebral (5, 7)	
	Strabismus (8)	
	Physiologic Nystagmus (8)	
	Spontaneous Nystagmus (8)	
	Mastication (5)	
	Facial Sensation (5)	
	Pinnae Sensation (7)	
	Tongue Tone (12)	
	Facial Muscle Symmetry (7)	
	Swallowing (9, 10)	

Hyperesthesia
Localization:_____

L	Superficial Pain (skin)	R
	Fore	
	Hind	

L	Deep Pain (bone)	R
	Fore	
	Hind	

Muscle Atrophy:_____

(1=hypo, 2=normal, 3=hyper)

L	Muscle Tone	R

L	Root Signature (holding limb up)	R

Modified Glasgow Coma Scale score:_____
(see page 190 for scoring instructions)

185

Neurological Examination

Patient:_____   **Date**:_____

- **Neurological History**:
  - ○ *Onset Date*:_____
  - ○ *Duration*:_____
  - ○ *Progression*: (*peracute / acute / chronic / progressive / static*)_____

- **Previous Treatments**:

Drug	Amount	Dose (mg/kg)	Route	Frequency	Duration

- ○ **Mental Status**:

Alert (conscious; responds to sensory stimuli)	Obtunded (↓ interaction w/ environment; slow response to verbal stimuli)	Stupor (unresponsive unless aroused by noxious stimuli)	Coma (complete unresponsiveness to any stimuli)

- ○ **Posture**:

Normal	Head Tilt (L / R)	Tremor	Falling	Circling (Tight / Wide) (L / R)

Schiff-Sherrington (rigid extension of forelimbs w/out forelimb paresis or ataxia)	Opisthotonus (backward arching of head, neck, and spine)	Decerebrate (opisthotonus + rigid extension of all limbs + stupor or coma)	Decerebellate (opisthotonus + rigid extension of fore-limbs + hip flexion + normal mentation)

- ○ **Gait**: *Affected Limb(s)*:

Ambulatory (able to stand and walk 10 steps unaided)		Non-ambulatory (unable to stand and walk 10 steps unaided)		
Normal	Paraparesis	Paraplegia	Tetraparesis	Tetraplegia
Monoparesis	Monoplegia	Hemiparesis	Hemiplegia	
Proprioceptive Ataxia		Cerebellar Ataxia		Vestib. Ataxia

- ○ **Motor**: Yes (voluntary movement)   No (absence of voluntary movement)

- ○ **Urination**: Yes (voluntary urination)   No (absence of voluntary urination)

(0=absent, 1=hypo, 2=normal)

L	Knuckling	R
	Front	
	Rear	

L	Hopping	R
	Front	
	Rear	

L	Ext. Post. Thrust	R
	Rear	

L	Wheelbarrowing	R
	Visual	
	Non-visual	

(0=absent, 1=hypo, 2=norm, 3=hyper, 4=clonus)

L	Nerve Function	R
	Biceps (C6-C8)	
	Triceps (C7-T1)	
	Extensor Carpi (C7-T1)	
	Withdrawal Forelimb (C6-T2)	
	Patellar (L4-L6)	
	Cranial Tibial (L6-L7)	
	Gastrocnemius (L6-S1)	
	Withdrawal Hindlimb (L5-S1)	
	Perineal (S1-S2)	
	Panniculus	
	Cross Extensor	
	Tail Tone	
	Anal Tone	

Neuroanatomical Localization
Generalized neuromuscular, Spinal cord (C1-C5), Spinal cord (C6-T2), Spinal cord (T3-L3), Spinal cord (L4-Cd5), Caudal brainstem, Cerebellum, Forebrain, Multifocal, Diffuse

(0=absent, 1=hypo, 2=normal)

L	Nerve Function	R
	Vision & Menace (2)	
	Pupil Size (2, 3)	
	Direct PLR (2, 3)	
	Indirect PLR (2, 3)	
	Palpebral (5, 7)	
	Strabismus (8)	
	Physiologic Nystagmus (8)	
	Spontaneous Nystagmus (8)	
	Mastication (5)	
	Facial Sensation (5)	
	Pinnae Sensation (7)	
	Tongue Tone (12)	
	Facial Muscle Symmetry (7)	
	Swallowing (9, 10)	

Hyperesthesia Localization:_____

L	Superficial Pain (skin)	R
	Fore	
	Hind	

L	Deep Pain (bone)	R
	Fore	
	Hind	

Muscle Atrophy:_____

(1=hypo, 2=normal, 3=hyper)

L	Muscle Tone	R

L	Root Signature (holding limb up)	R

Modified Glasgow Coma Scale score:_____
(see page 190 for scoring instructions)

Neurological Examination

Patient:_____ **Date**:_____

- **Neurological History**:
    - *Onset Date*:_____
    - *Duration*:_____
    - *Progression*: (*peracute / acute / chronic / progressive / static*)_____

- **Previous Treatments**:

Drug	Amount	Dose (mg/kg)	Route	Frequency	Duration

- ○ *Mental Status*:

Alert (conscious; responds to sensory stimuli)	Obtunded (↓ interaction w/ environment; slow response to verbal stimuli)	Stupor (unresponsive unless aroused by noxious stimuli)	Coma (complete unresponsiveness to any stimuli)

- ○ *Posture*:

Normal	Head Tilt (L / R)	Tremor	Falling	Circling (Tight / Wide) (L / R)
Schiff-Sherrington (rigid extension of forelimbs w/out forelimb paresis or ataxia)	Opisthotonus (backward arching of head, neck, and spine)	Decerebrate (opisthotonus + rigid extension of all limbs + stupor or coma)	Decerebellate (opisthotonus + rigid extension of fore-limbs + hip flexion + normal mentation)	

- ○ *Gait*: *Affected Limb(s)*:

Ambulatory (able to stand and walk 10 steps unaided)		Non-ambulatory (unable to stand and walk 10 steps unaided)		
Normal	Paraparesis	Paraplegia	Tetraparesis	Tetraplegia
Monoparesis	Monoplegia	Hemiparesis	Hemiplegia	
Proprioceptive Ataxia		Cerebellar Ataxia		Vestib. Ataxia

- ○ *Motor*: Yes (voluntary movement)   No (absence of voluntary movement)

- ○ *Urination*: Yes (voluntary urination)   No (absence of voluntary urination)

(0=absent, 1=hypo, 2=normal)

L	Knuckling	R
	Front	
	Rear	

L	Hopping	R
	Front	
	Rear	

L	Ext. Post. Thrust	R
	Rear	

L	Wheelbarrowing	R
	Visual	
	Non-visual	

(0=absent, 1=hypo, 2=norm, 3=hyper, 4=clonus)

L	Nerve Function	R
	Biceps (C6-C8)	
	Triceps (C7-T1)	
	Extensor Carpi (C7-T1)	
	Withdrawal Forelimb (C6-T2)	
	Patellar (L4-L6)	
	Cranial Tibial (L6-L7)	
	Gastrocnemius (L6-S1)	
	Withdrawal Hindlimb (L5-S1)	
	Perineal (S1-S2)	
	Panniculus	
	Cross Extensor	
	Tail Tone	
	Anal Tone	

Neuroanatomical Localization
Generalized neuromuscular, Spinal cord (C1-C5), Spinal cord (C6-T2), Spinal cord (T3-L3), Spinal cord (L4-Cd5), Caudal brainstem, Cerebellum, Forebrain, Multifocal, Diffuse

(0=absent, 1=hypo, 2=normal)

L	Nerve Function	R
	Vision & Menace (2)	
	Pupil Size (2, 3)	
	Direct PLR (2, 3)	
	Indirect PLR (2, 3)	
	Palpebral (5, 7)	
	Strabismus (8)	
	Physiologic Nystagmus (8)	
	Spontaneous Nystagmus (8)	
	Mastication (5)	
	Facial Sensation (5)	
	Pinnae Sensation (7)	
	Tongue Tone (12)	
	Facial Muscle Symmetry (7)	
	Swallowing (9, 10)	

Hyperesthesia Localization:_____

L	Superficial Pain (skin)	R
	Fore	
	Hind	

L	Deep Pain (bone)	R
	Fore	
	Hind	

Muscle Atrophy:_____

(1=hypo, 2=normal, 3=hyper)

L	Muscle Tone	R

L	Root Signature (holding limb up)	R

Modified Glasgow Coma Scale score:_____
(see page 190 for scoring instructions)

Modified Glasgow Coma Scale (MGCS)

		Score
Motor Activity	Normal gait, normal spinal reflexes	6
	Hemiparesis, tetraparesis, or decerebrate rigidity	5
	Recumbent, intermittent extensor rigidity	4
	Recumbent, constant extensor rigidity	3
	Recumbent, constant extensor rigidity w/ opisthotonus	2
	Recumbent, hypotonia of muscles, depressed or absent spinal reflexes	1
Brainstem Reflexes	Normal pupillary light reflexes and oculocephalic reflexes	6
	Slow pupillary light reflexes and normal to reduced oculocephalic reflexes	5
	Bilateral unresponsive miosis w/ normal to reduced oculocephalic reflexes	4
	Pinpoint pupils w/ reduced to absent oculocephalic reflexes	3
	Unilateral, unresponsive mydriasis w/ reduced to absent oculocephalic reflexes	2
	Bilateral, unresponsive mydriasis w/ reduced to absent oculocephalic reflexes	1
Level of Consciousness	Occasional periods of alertness and responsive to environment	6
	Depression or delirium, capable of responding but response may be inappropriate	5
	Semicomatose, responsive to visual stimuli	4
	Semicomatose, responsive to auditory stimuli	3
	Semicomatose, responsive only to repeated noxious stimuli	2
	Comatose, unresponsive to repeated noxious stimuli	1

Interpretation of MGCS Score

The *Modified Glasgow Coma Scale (MGCS)* is an objective way to evaluate neurologic function of dogs after traumatic brain injury. The score is a useful way to monitor progression of neurologic deficits, effects of therapeutic measures, and to assess overall prognosis.

Application:
- When possible, the initial neurological examination (including MGCS scale scoring) should occur before any analgesic therapy to allow adequate assessment of the neurologic status.
- Resuscitation is also necessary prior to the neuro exam because shock can affect neurologic status.
- Repeated neurological assessment is recommended every 30–60 minutes after initial presentation and after interventions are made.

Predicting Prognosis

3-8	Grave
9-14	Guarded
15-18	Good

Other Specific Numbers From Literature

8	50% mortality within the first 48 hours of traumatic brain injury
≤17	Sensitivity of 82% and a specificity of 87% for predicting non-survival to hospital discharge

• Source: *Textbook of Small Animal Emergency*, First Edition. Edited by Kenneth J. Drobatz, Kate Hopper, Elizabeth Rozanski, and Deborah C. Silverstein. © 2019 John Wiley & Sons, Inc.

Ophthalmology Examination

Patient: _____   **Date:** _____

- **Ophthalmic History:**
  - *Onset Date:* _____
  - *Duration:* _____
  - *Progression:* (*peracute / acute / chronic / progressive / static*) _____

OD	Minimum Database	OS
	Menace	
	Dazzle	
	Direct PLR	
	Indirect PLR	
	Tapetal reflection	
	Palpebral reflex	
	± Corneal reflex	
	Oculocephalic reflex	
	Retropulsion	
	Schirmer TT (>15 mm/min)*	
	Fluorescein stain uptake	
	Seidel test (+=corneal perf.)	
	Tonometry (10–20 mmHg)§	
	± Photopic maze (in light)	
	± Scotopic maze (in dark)	
	Aqueous flare (0-4)	

Lesions on Extraocular Exam and Fundoscopy	
Keratitis	Superficial corneal neovascularization
	Corneal fibrosis
	Superficial corneal pigmentation
	Corneal ulceration
Conjunct-ivitis	Mucoid to mucopurulent discharge
	Blepharospasm
	Epiphora
	Conjunctival hyperemia
	Conjunctival lymphoid follicles
	Chemosis
Uveitis	Aqueous flare (pathognomonic)
	Keratic precipitates (pathognomonic)
	Hypopyon, hyphema, fibrin (pathognomonic)
	Miosis
	Retinal hemorrhage or hyporeflectivity
Glaucoma	Episcleral injection
	Blepharospasm
	Corneal edema
	Mydriasis
	Optic disc cupping
	Buphthalmos (enlargement of globe)
	Lens (sub)luxation (common in terriers)
Lens Opacity	Nuclear sclerosis (bluish-gray haziness of lens nucleus; tapetal reflection and fundus visible through opacity)
	Cataract (tapetal reflection not visible through opacity); (<20%=incipient; 20–100%= incomplete; 100%=complete)
Other	Exophthalmos (protrusion + normal size)
	Proptosis (protrusion + eyelids caught behind globe equator)

*Tonometry:
- Lowest reading is most accurate.
- Coefficient of variance should be 95% or 5% based on device.
- <10 mmHg = consistent with uveitis or chronic glaucoma.
- ≥25 mmHg = diagnostic for glaucoma (especially if blind).
- ≥50 mmHg = pressures at which blindness occurs.
- *Contraindications:* ocular trauma (ex., ruptured globe), corneal abrasion or ulcer (do not touch lesion with tonometer), inability to apply topical anesthetics (proparacaine); perform before pupil dilation (tropicamide).

§Schirmer Tear Test:
- <15 mm/min + clinical signs = diagnostic for quantitative KCS.
- ≥15 mm/min + clinical signs = diagnostic for qualitative KCS.
- Clinical signs of KCS are those of keratitis and conjunctivitis.
- *Contraindications:* not performed in cats, deep corneal ulcer, descemetocele, corneal perforation; not necessary with epiphora; perform before any drops or sedation.

Ophthalmology Examination

Patient:_____   **Date**:_____

- **Ophthalmic History**:
  - *Onset Date*:_____
  - *Duration*:_____
  - *Progression*: (*peracute / acute / chronic / progressive / static*)_____

OD	Minimum Database	OS
	Menace	
	Dazzle	
	Direct PLR	
	Indirect PLR	
	Tapetal reflection	
	Palpebral reflex	
	± Corneal reflex	
	Oculocephalic reflex	
	Retropulsion	
	Schirmer TT (>15 mm/min)*	
	Fluorescein stain uptake	
	Seidel test (+=corneal perf.)	
	Tonometry (10–20 mmHg)§	
	± Photopic maze (in light)	
	± Scotopic maze (in dark)	
	Aqueous flare (0-4)	

*Tonometry:
- Lowest reading is most accurate.
- Coefficient of variance should be 95% or 5% based on device.
- <10 mmHg = consistent with uveitis or chronic glaucoma.
- ≥25 mmHg = diagnostic for glaucoma (especially if blind).
- ≥50 mmHg = pressures at which blindness occurs.
- *Contraindications*: ocular trauma (ex., ruptured globe), corneal abrasion or ulcer (do not touch lesion with tonometer), inability to apply topical anesthetics (proparacaine); perform before pupil dilation (tropicamide).

§**Schirmer Tear Test**:
- <15 mm/min + clinical signs = diagnostic for quantitative KCS.
- ≥15 mm/min + clinical signs = diagnostic for qualitative KCS.
- Clinical signs of KCS are those of keratitis and conjunctivitis.
- *Contraindications*: not performed in cats, deep corneal ulcer, descemetocele, corneal perforation; not necessary with epiphora; perform before any drops or sedation.

Lesions on Extraocular Exam and Fundoscopy	
Keratitis	Superficial corneal neovascularization
	Corneal fibrosis
	Superficial corneal pigmentation
	Corneal ulceration
Conjunct-ivitis	Mucoid to mucopurulent discharge
	Blepharospasm
	Epiphora
	Conjunctival hyperemia
	Conjunctival lymphoid follicles
	Chemosis
Uveitis	Aqueous flare (pathognomonic)
	Keratic precipitates (pathognomonic)
	Hypopyon, hyphema, fibrin (pathognomonic)
	Miosis
	Retinal hemorrhage or hyporeflectivity
Glaucoma	Episcleral injection
	Blepharospasm
	Corneal edema
	Mydriasis
	Optic disc cupping
	Buphthalmos (enlargement of globe)
	Lens (sub)luxation (common in terriers)
Lens Opacity	Nuclear sclerosis (bluish-gray haziness of lens nucleus; tapetal reflection and fundus visible through opacity)
	Cataract (tapetal reflection not visible through opacity); (<20%=incipient; 20–100%= incomplete; 100%=complete)
Other	Exophthalmos (protrusion + normal size)
	Proptosis (protrusion + eyelids caught behind globe equator)

Ophthalmology Examination

Patient:_____   **Date**:_____

- **Ophthalmic History**:
  - *Onset Date*:_____
  - *Duration*:_____
  - *Progression*: (*peracute / acute / chronic / progressive / static*)_____

OD	*Minimum Database*	OS
	Menace	
	Dazzle	
	Direct PLR	
	Indirect PLR	
	Tapetal reflection	
	Palpebral reflex	
	± Corneal reflex	
	Oculocephalic reflex	
	Retropulsion	
	Schirmer TT (>15 mm/min)*	
	Fluorescein stain uptake	
	Seidel test (+=corneal perf.)	
	Tonometry (10–20 mmHg)§	
	± Photopic maze (in light)	
	± Scotopic maze (in dark)	
	Aqueous flare (0-4)	

Lesions on Extraocular Exam and Fundoscopy	
Keratitis	Superficial corneal neovascularization
	Corneal fibrosis
	Superficial corneal pigmentation
	Corneal ulceration
Conjunct-ivitis	Mucoid to mucopurulent discharge
	Blepharospasm
	Epiphora
	Conjunctival hyperemia
	Conjunctival lymphoid follicles
	Chemosis
Uveitis	Aqueous flare (pathognomonic)
	Keratic precipitates (pathognomonic)
	Hypopyon, hyphema, fibrin (pathognomonic)
	Miosis
	Retinal hemorrhage or hyporeflectivity
Glaucoma	Episcleral injection
	Blepharospasm
	Corneal edema
	Mydriasis
	Optic disc cupping
	Buphthalmos (enlargement of globe)
	Lens (sub)luxation (common in terriers)
Lens Opacity	Nuclear sclerosis (bluish-gray haziness of lens nucleus; tapetal reflection and fundus visible through opacity)
	Cataract (tapetal reflection not visible through opacity); (<20%=incipient; 20–100%= incomplete; 100%=complete)
Other	Exophthalmos (protrusion + normal size)
	Proptosis (protrusion + eyelids caught behind globe equator)

*Tonometry:
- Lowest reading is most accurate.
- Coefficient of variance should be 95% or 5% based on device.
- <10 mmHg = consistent with uveitis or chronic glaucoma.
- ≥25 mmHg = diagnostic for glaucoma (especially if blind).
- ≥50 mmHg = pressures at which blindness occurs.
- *Contraindications*: ocular trauma (ex., ruptured globe), corneal abrasion or ulcer (do not touch lesion with tonometer), inability to apply topical anesthetics (proparacaine); perform before pupil dilation (tropicamide).

§Schirmer Tear Test:
- <15 mm/min + clinical signs = diagnostic for quantitative KCS.
- ≥15 mm/min + clinical signs = diagnostic for qualitative KCS.
- Clinical signs of KCS are those of keratitis and conjunctivitis.
- *Contraindications*: not performed in cats, deep corneal ulcer, descemetocele, corneal perforation; not necessary with epiphora; perform before any drops or sedation.

Sources Cited:

1. *IRIS Staging of CKD*. © 2017 International Renal Interest Society (IRIS) Ltd.

2. Prittie, J. (2006). Optimal endpoints of resuscitation and early goal-directed therapy. *Journal of Veterinary Emergency and Critical Care, 16*(4), 329-339. doi:10.1111/j.1476-4431.2006.00160.x

3. *Shock Pathophysiology*. Edited by Elizabeth Thomovsky and Paula A. Johnson. © 2013 Vetstreet, Inc.

4. *Small Animal Clinical Diagnosis by Laboratory Methods*, Fifth Edition. Edited by Michael D. Willard and Harold Tvedten. © 2012 Saunders.

5. *Textbook of Small Animal Emergency*, First Edition. Edited by Kenneth J. Drobatz, Kate Hopper, Elizabeth Rozanski, and Deborah C. Silverstein. © 2019 John Wiley & Sons, Inc.

"Because you are alive, everything is possible."
- *Thich Nhat Hanh*

Physical Examination Findings at Each Stage of Shock						
	DOG			CAT		
	Compensated Shock	Acute Decompensated Shock	Late Decompensated Shock	Compensated Shock	Acute Decompensated Shock	Late Decompensated Shock
Temp. (°F)	↓ (98–99)	↓↓ (96–98)	↓↓↓ (<96)	↓ (<97)	↓↓ (<95)	↓↓↓ (<90)
HR (bpm)	↑↑ (>180)	↑ (>150)	↓-to-N (<140)	↑↑↑ (>240) ↓ (160–180)	↑↑ (>200) ↓↓ (120–140)	↑ (>180) ↓↓↓ (<120)
RR (rpm)	↑↑ (>50)	↑ (<50)	N-↑-Agonal	↑↑↑ (>60)	↑↑ (>60)	↑-to-Agonal
Mentation	QAR	Obtunded	Obtunded-to-Stupor	QAR	Obtunded	Obtunded-to-Stupor
MM color	Pale	Pale	Pale-to-Muddy	Pale	Pale-to-White	Pale-to-White
CRT (sec)	< 1	< 2	≥ 2	< 1	< 2	≥ 2
MAP (mm Hg)	↓-to-N (70–80)	↓ (50–70)	↓↓ (<60)	↓-to-N (80–90)	↓ (50–80)	↓↓ (<50)

- Source: 3

Endpoints of Resuscitation	
Mentation	Normal
Heart Rate	Dog: 70–140; Cat: 140–180 (stressed: 180–220)
Blood Pressure	SAP >90 mmHg; MAP >60 mmHg
Lactate	< 2 mmol/L

- Source: 2

Fluid Therapy			
	Hydration		
Resuscitation	Fluid Deficit / Dehydration	Maintenance	Ongoing Losses

• Traditional "shock dose":
  ◦ **Dog = ¼ of 90 ml/kg** (over 15 min)
 	
  ◦ **Cat = ¼ of 60 ml/kg** (over 15 min)
 	
• Reevaluate based on endpoints of resuscitation.
	• **Liters of dehydration = (kg) × (% dehydration)**
	
	• Subtract shock bolus volumes from fluid deficit.
	
	• Replace over 6–24 hour depending on patient.
	
	• Example:
	  ◦ BW = 11 kg
	  ◦ Estimated Dehydration = 7%
	  ◦ Fluid deficit = (11)(0.07) = 0.77L = 770mL
		• Traditional formulas:
		  ◦ **Dog = 40–60 ml/kg/day**
		
		  ◦ **Cat = 48–72 ml/kg/day**
		
		  ◦ **Pediatric = 80–120 ml/kg/day**
		
		• Accounts for daily fluid losses from feces, skin, breathing, urine.
			• Replace measured volumes of:
			  ◦ Vomit
			  ◦ Regurg.
			  ◦ Diarrhea
			  ◦ Saliva
			  ◦ Blood loss
			  ◦ Draining fluid

- Subcutaneous fluid dose (outpatient treatment of dehydration with mild clinical signs and normal tissue perfusion parameters): 10–30 mL/kg
- Source: 5

Reference Intervals

CBC:

- **RBC** ($10^6/\mu l$): *D-RI*: 5.5-8.5; *C-RI*: 5-10
- **PCV** (%): *D-RI*: 37-56; *C-RI*: 24-45
  - *Mild Anemia*: D30 –37; C20–26
  - *Moderate Anemia*: D20–29; C14–19
  - *Severe Anemia*: D13–19; C10–13
  - *Very Severe Anemia*: D<13; C<10
  - *Anemia of Chronic Disease*: D25–35; C20–25 (normocytic, normochromic)
- **HGB** (g/dl): *D-RI*: 10-20; *C-RI*: 8-15
- **MCV** (fL): *D-RI*: 60-77; *C-RI*: 39-55
- **MCHC** (g/dl): *D-RI*: 32-36; *C-RI*: 31-35
- **RETIC** (/μl): *D-Regen*: ≥60,000; *C-Regen*: ≥50,000 aggregate
- **WBC** ($10^3/\mu l$): *D-RI*: 6-17; *C-RI*: 5.5-19
  - *Leukemoid Reaction*: >50,000–100,000 /μl (without leukemia)
- **NEU** ($10^3/\mu l$): *D-RI*: 3-11.5; *C-RI*: 2.5-12.5
  - *Corticosteroid Response*: ~15,000–25,000 /μl (<40,000 /μl)
  - *Require Sepsis Monitoring*: <1,000–2,000 /μl
  - *Presumed Sepsis*: <500–1,000 /μl and febrile
  - *Suspend Chemotherapy with Myelosuppressive Agents*: <2,500 /μl
- **BAND** (/μl): *DC-RI*: 0-300
  - *Inflammatory Disease*: neutrophilia with a left shift >1,000 non-seg/μl
- **LYM** ($10^3/\mu l$): *D-RI*: 1-4.8; *C-RI*: 1.5-7
- **MONO** (/μl): *D-RI*: 150-1250; *C-RI*: 0-850
- **EOS** (/μl): *D-RI*: 100-1250; *C-RI*: 0-1500
- **BASO** (/μl): *DC-RI*: 0-150
- **PLT** ($10^3/\mu l$): *D-RI*: 200-500; *C-RI*: 300-800; *Greyhound Dogs*: ~150
  - *Risk of Spontaneous Thrombosis*: >1,000,000 /μl
  - *Risk of DIC*: >50,000 /μl and patient is spontaneously bleeding
  - *Risk of Spontaneous Bleed*: <30,000–50,000 /μl
  - *Top Differential is IMT*: <50,000 /μl
  - *Suspend Chemotherapy with Myelosuppressive Agents*: <50,000 /μl
  - *Normal Cavalier King Charles Spaniel & Norfolk Terrier*: <10,000 /μl
- **TS-Plasma** (g/dl): *DC-RI*: 6-8

Urinalysis:

- **USG** (GMS/1000): *Dog-RI*: ≥1.030; *Cat-RI*: ≥1.035
- **PH**: *DC-RI*: 6.0-7.0
- **Protein** (mg/dl): *D-RI*: 0-30 or trace with USG >1.012; *C-RI*: Neg
- **Glucose** (mg/dl): *DC-RI*: Neg
- **Ketones**: *DC-RI*: Neg
- **Bilirubin**: *D-RI*: Neg or trace with USG ≥1.030; *C-RI*: Neg
- **SSA** (protein): *D-RI*: 1+ with USG >1.012; *C-RI*: Neg
- **Acetest** (ketone): *DC-RI*: Neg
- **Ictotest** (bilirub): *D-RI*: Neg or trace with USG ≥1.030; *C-RI*: Neg
- **Casts** (/lpf): *DC-RI*: 0-2 hyaline or granular casts
- **WBC** (/hpf): *DC-RI*: <4
- **RBC** (/hpf): *DC-RI*: <5
- **Bacteria**: *DC-RI*: Neg in cysto sample
- **Cells** (/hpf): *DC-RI*: 0-2
- **Crystals**: *DC-RI*: None to Few
- **Urine Protein/Creatinine Ratio (U/PC)**:
  - *Non-proteinuric*: D<0.2; C<0.2
  - *Borderline proteinuric*: D0.2-0.5; C0.2-0.4
  - *Proteinuric*: D>0.5; C<0.4

Venous Blood Gas:
- **pH**: *D-RI*: 7.32-7.40; *C-RI*: 7.28-7.41; (7.1<☘>7.6)
- **PCO2** (mm Hg): *D-RI*: 33-50; *C-RI*: 33-45
- **HCO3** (mEq/L): *D-RI*: 18-26; *C-RI*: 18-23

Arterial Blood Gas:
- **pH**: *D-RI*: 7.36-7.44; *C-RI*: 7.36-7.44; (7.1<☘>7.6)
- **PCO2** (mm Hg): *D-RI*: 36-44; *C-RI*: 28-32; (☘>70)
- **HCO3** (mEq/L): *D-RI*: 18-26; *C-RI*: 17-22
- PO2 (mm Hg): *D-RI*: ≈100; *C-RI*: ≈100; (☘<60)

Serum Biochemistry:

- **Glucose** (mg/dl): *D-RI*: 60-135; *C-RI*: 65-131; (40<☠>1000)
  - *Coma or Seizures*: <40; *Hyperosmotic diabetes with CNS dysfunction*: >1,000
- **Lactic Acid** (mg/dl): *D-RI*: 9.9-46.8; *C-RI*: 5.4-15.3
  - Lactic Acid (mmol/L): *DC-RI*: 0.22-1.44; (☠>6.0; associated with a poor prognosis)
- **Cholesterol** (mg/dl): *D-RI*: 120-247; *C-RI*: 56-161
- **SDMA** (μg/dl): *DC-RI*: 0-14
- **BUN** (mg/dl): *D-RI*: 5-29; *C-RI*: 19-33
- **Creatinine** (mg/dl): *D-RI*: 0.3-2; *C-RI*: 0.8-1.8
- **Na** (mmol/l): *D-RI*: 139-147; *C-RI*: 144-155; (120<☠>170)
  - *CNS signs*: <120 or >170 in dogs
- **K** (mmol/l): *D-RI*: 3.3-4.6; *C-RI*: 3.5-5.1; (2.5<☠>7.5)
  - *Muscle weakness*: <2.5; *Cardiac conduction disturbances*: >7.5
- **Cl** (mEq/l): *D-RI*: 107-116; *C-RI*: 113-123
- **Na:K Ratio**: *Addison's suspect at* <27:1
- **Total Ca** (mg/dl): *D-RI*: 9.3-11.8; *C-RI*: 8.4-11.8; (7.0<☠>16)
  - *Tetany*: <7.0; *Acute renal failure and cardiac toxicity*: >16
- **Ionized Ca** (mmol/L): *DC-RI*: 1.12-1.42
- **P** (mg/dl): *D-RI*: 2.9-6.2; *C-RI*: 3.8-7.5; (☠ <1.5)
  - *Hemolysis, CNS signs*: <1.5
- **Ca×P Product** (mg/dL): *Mineralization at* >60
- **Mg** (mg/dl): *D-RI*: 1.7-2.1; *C-RI*: 1.7-2.3 (1<☠>10)
- **HCO3** (mmol/l): *D-RI*: 21-28; *C-RI*: 19-26 (☠ <12)
  - *Suspect severe metabolic acidosis*: <12
- **AG** (mmol/l): *D-RI*: 10-18; *C-RI*: 12-19
- **OSM** (mOsm/kg): *D-RI*: 290-310; *C-RI*: 308-335
- **TP** (g/dl): *D-RI*: 5.7-7.8; *C-RI*: 6.1-7.7
- **Albumin** (g/dl): *D-RI*: 2.4-3.6; *C-RI*: 2.5-3.3; (☠ ≤1.5)
  - *Severe hypoalbuminemia; at risk for major fluid shifts*: ≤1.5
- **Globulin** (g/dl): *D-RI*: 1.7-3.8; *C-RI*: 2.3-3.8
  - *Severe hyperglobulinemia*: ≥5
- **Bilirubin** (mg/dl): *D-RI*: 0-0.8; *C-RI*: 0-0.6
  - *Icteric plasma*: ≥1.5; *Icteric mucous membranes*: ≥3
- **ALT** (U/L): *D-RI*: 10-130; *C-RI*: 26-84
- **ALP** (U/L): *D-RI*: 24-147; *C-RI*: 20-109
- **GGT** (U/L): *D-RI*: 0-25; *C-RI*: 0-12

Other Diagnostics:

- **Systolic Blood Pressure** (mm Hg): *DC-RI*:
  - *Hypo*: <80; *Normo*: 90–140; *Prehyper*: 140–159; *Hyper*: 160–179; *Severely Hyper*: ≥180
- **Mean Arterial Blood Pressure** (mm Hg): *DC-RI*: 60–100
- **Central Venous Pressure** (mm Hg): *DC-RI*: 3–8
- **SpO2** (Pulse Oximetry – hemoglobin saturation with oxygen) (%): *DC-RI*: ≥95
- **ETCO2** (Capnography – an estimate of PaCO2) (mm Hg): *DC-RI*: 35–45
- **BMBT** (min): *Normal platelet function in D*: 2.6 ± 0.5
- **D-Dimer** (μg/ml):
  - <0.25 has a strong NPV to (more or less) rule out DIC
  - >0.5 is characteristic for PTE in dogs (Se 100%; Sp 70%)
- **T4** (μg/dl): *D-RI*: 0.8-3.5; *C-RI*: 1-4
- **Cortisol** (μg/dl): *D-RI*: 1-6; *C-RI*: 1-5
  - *Addison's suspect*: <2 (must perform ACTH-stimulation test)

- *Key: D* – dog; *C* – cat; *RI* – reference interval; *Regen* – regenerative; *Neg* – negative; ☠ – danger values
- *Helpful Equations*:
  - **RETIC (/μl)** = (RETIC[%]) × (RBC [10^6/μl])
  - **Corrected WBC count** = (NRBC × 100) / (NRBC + 100) [calculate if if nRBCs are >5]
  - **Corrected Total Serum Calcium** = tCa (mg/dl) – Alb (g/dl) + 3.5 [Calculate if ↓ alb]
  - **AG** = [Na + K] – [Cl + HCO3]
  - **OSM (Osmolality)** = 1.86(Na + K) + (BUN/2.8) + (Glucose/18) + 9
  - **Osmol Gap** = measured OSM – calculated OSM [>25 mOsm/kg = presence of unmeasured osmols]
- *Sources*: 1, 4, 5; most CBC and serum biochemistry reference interval data are provided by the in-house Small Animal Clinical Pathology lab at the Texas A&M University Veterinary Medical Teaching Hospital

Emergency Drug Doses

Drug	Canine Dose	Feline Dose
Acepromazine	0.01–0.2 mg/kg, IV/ IM/ SC (max. 3 mg)	0.01–0.2 mg/kg, IV/ IM/ SC (max. 1 mg)
Apomorphine	0.03 mg/kg, IV (for emesis); 0.04 mg/kg, IM (for emesis); 0.02 mg/kg, SC (for emesis); 1.5–6 mg, in conjunctival sac (for emesis);	–
Atipamezole	3750 μg/m² BSA, IM (to reverse α2-agonists); 0.1 mg/kg, IV (to reverse α2-agonist in CPR)	Same
Atropine sulfate	0.04 mg/kg, IV/ IM/ IO (for CPR or atropine response test); 0.15–0.2 mg/kg, diluted 1:10 in saline or water, Intratrach	Same
Buprenorphine	0.005–0.03 mg/kg, IV/ IM/ SC, q6–12h; 0.12 mg/kg, Oral Transmucosal	0.01–0.03 mg/kg, IV/ IM, q6–8h; 0.03 mg/kg, Oral Transmucosal, q6–8h
Butorphanol	0.1–0.5 mg/kg, IV/ IM/ SC, q1–4h	0.1–0.5 mg/kg, IV/ IM/ SC, q1–4h
Butorphanol +Dexmedetomidine ± Ketamine	Butorphanol 0.4 mg/kg + Dexmedetomidine 0.005–0.01 mg/kg, mix in same syringe and give IM (if no evidence of cardiovascular disease)	Butorphanol 0.3 mg/kg + Dexmedetomidine 0.005–0.01 mg/kg ± Ketamine 3 mg/kg, mix in same syringe and give IM (duration of sedation is longer when ketamine is added)
Butorphanol +Midazolam +Other	Butorphanol 0.2 mg/kg, IV + Midazolam 0.2 mg/kg, IV + Alfaxalone 2 mg/kg, IV over 1 minute (provides excellent induction and recovery with minimal cardiopulmonary effects)	Butorphanol 0.4 mg/kg + Midazolam 0.4 mg/kg + Ketamine 3 mg/kg, mix in same syringe and give IM (provides good sedation for physiologically-compromised cats)
Calcium gluconate (10%)	1 mL/kg of 10% solution (which corresponds to 100 mg/kg of calcium gluconate), IV slowly over 10–20 min (for treatment of hyperkalemia with K⁺ >8 mEq/L)	Same
Dexamethasone	0.07–0.14 mg/kg/day (anti-inflammatory), IV/ IM/ SC	Same
Dexmedetomidine	0.001–0.005 mg/kg, IV (or 125–375 μg/m² BSA, IV); 0.001–0.02 mg/kg, IM (or 165–500 μg/m² BSA, IM)	Same
Dextrose (50%)	0.5–1 mL/kg (0.25–0.5 g/kg), diluted 1:2 in sterile saline or water, IV slowly over 5 min (for treatment of hypoglycemia)	Same
Diazepam	0.5–2 mg/kg, IV/ Rectal/ Intranasal (for status epilepticus)	Same
Diphenhydramine	0.5–2 mg/kg, IV/ IM, q8–12h; 2–4 mg/kg, PO, q8–12h	Same
Epinephrine	0.01 mg/kg, IV/ IO, q3–5min in early CPR (low dose); 0.1 mg/kg, IV/ IO, q3–5min in prolonged CPR (high dose) * *1:1000=1 mg/mL; 1:10,000=0.1 mg/mL*	Same
Flumazenil	0.01 mg/kg, IV/ IO, q1h as needed (to reverse benzodiazepines)	Same
Furosemide	1–4 mg/kg, IV/ IM/ SC, q1–2h	2–4 mg/kg, IV/ IM/ SC, q1–2h

Drug	Canine Dose	Feline Dose
Hydromorphone	0.05–0.2 mg/kg, IV/ IM/ SC, q2–4h (for analgesia)	0.05–0.1 mg/kg, IV/ IM/ SC, q2–6h
HES 6%	10–20 mL/kg, IV, given over 15–30 min (shock bolus)	5–10 mL/kg, IV, given over 15–30 min (shock bolus)
Hypertonic saline (7–7.5% NaCl)	4–5 mL/kg, IV, given over 5–10 min	3–4 mL/kg, IV, given over 5–10 min
Lidocaine[†]	2 mg/kg, IV, given over 2 min (for ventricular arrhythmia)	0.25–0.5 mg/kg, IV, given over 5 min (for ventricular arrhythmia)
Mannitol	0.5–1 g/kg, IV, given over 10–20 min, q6h	Same
Methadone	0.1–1 mg/kg, IV/ IM/ SC, q4–8h (for analgesia)	0.05–0.5 mg/kg, IV/ IM/ SC, q4–6h (for analgesia)
Midazolam	0.1–0.3 mg/kg, IV/ IM/ Intranasal (for status epilepticus)	Same
Morphine	0.5–1 mg/kg, IV/ IM/ SC, given over 2 min, q2h (for analgesia)	0.05–0.4 mg/kg, IM/ SC, q3h (for analgesia)
Naloxone	0.01–0.04 mg/kg, IV/ IM/ SC/ IO (to reverse opioid)	Same
Packed RBCs	10 mL/kg, IV (1 mL/kg to raise PCV 1%)	Same
Plasma	6–20 mL/kg, IV, PRN for coagulopathy	Same
Prednisolone	0.5–1 mg/kg/day (anti-inflammatory), IV/ PO	Same
Procainamide	2 mg/kg, IV, given over 3–5 min, up to a total dose of 20 mg/kg (for atrial or ventricular arrhythmia)	–
Propofol	2–6 mg/kg, IV slowly to effect	Same
Terbutaline	–	0.01 mg/kg, IV/ IM/ SC, q4h (for asthma)
Whole blood	10–20 mL/kg, IV (2 mL/kg to raise PCV 1%)	Same
Xylazine	–	0.4–1.1 mg/kg, IV/ IM/ SC (for emesis)

† *Clinically-significant ventricular tachycardia*: ≥4 ventricular premature complexes consecutively at a rate of ≥160 bpm in dogs (≥240 bpm in cats)
   • Sources: 3, 8, 11